MW00571609

Introduction

In 1969 a little Korean woman stood on the platform of a train and looked back at her family, her children, her homeland before turning to a new life in a new world. *Passing the Torch,* written as a series of letters, is the remarkable story of that little woman, Doctor Chi Sun Rhee.

In 1933, when Doctor Rhee was born, the Japanese controlled Korea, and she learned her first lessons at school in the Japanese language. In 1956, when she begins her story, the wheel of history had turned—Korea was beginning to recover from the brutality of two wars, and the 5000-year-old traditions of that ancient land were changing. Chi Sun Rhee was at the forefront of those changes—an educated woman, a teacher in a culture that expected a woman to marry at seventeen and to devote her life only to her family. Chi Sun says that she felt called to a "shining greatness," and this book, written for her daughter, tells of her struggle to reach her own potential while conforming in many ways to the expectations of her family. She allowed her family to arrange her marriage, yes—but she chose the one man among the proposed suitors who would encourage her to have her own career. Her wedding was conducted according to ancient tradition, her first visit to her husband's family followed prescribed rites, her first baby was born with only her mother-in-law in attendance. But she took advantage of the new opportunities in society—she kept her job after her first baby arrived, she entered medical school when that child was three, she graduated with honors, she had two more children but completed her residency in obstetrics and gynecology in Korea.

When her husband decided to come to America for graduate work in political science, she came with him, leaving her three children in Korea for a year with her mother. She completed another four-year residency in this country; during that time, she brought her children here, where they started school immediately although they spoke no English. Doctor Rhee practiced medicine in Monroe, Michigan until her retirement in 1986. She and John became American citizens, settled in Toledo, Ohio, where John is President of the Korean Society of Greater Toledo, and raised their children as Americans. And all three of those little children who couldn't speak English grew up to be medical doctors.

Passing the Torch can be read on several levels. First, it is a wonderful love story. John Rhee is a remarkable man—one who not only allowed Chi Sun to follow her dream but who made that dream come true. He put her through medical school, supported her both financially and emotionally through the stress of training, accepted her long hours away from home, and glowed with genuine pride at her achievements. This is a portrait of a strong, inviolable marriage. On another level, it is a marvelously detailed picture of a culture that Americans know little about. It tells in exotic and colorful detail of the matchmakers who bring together lifelong partners, the elaborate Korean wedding ceremony, the traditional visit of a bride to the family of her husband, the customs surrounding the birth of a Korean baby.

On still another level, this is the story of the making of a doctor, with vivid descriptions of the operating room, the first delivery of a baby from a doctor's perspective, the long night vigils of a dedicated obstetrician, the case histories of women at the beginning and at the end of life. And on still another level, it is the story of the struggle of sensitive people to adapt to utterly foreign conventions—the confrontation with prejudice, the difficulty with language, the differences in clothing and in mores and in manners.

And finally, and most important, this is a glimpse into the soul of a poet. For everything that Chi Sun writes about is radiant, glowing in color and insight and metaphor. Her ability to paint a picture shines through passages such as this, when she leaves Korea for America and presses her face against the train window for the last sight of her homeland:

> The ranges of endless mountains, rank on rank, the green pines, the plains wide or narrow—they symbolize our land and people who are ever strong, stately, and young like them. The rice plants of darkest green cover the expanse of the plains; in the distance a band of farmers in white—wearing long pants rolled up to the knees and wide-brimmed straw hats—are working in the rice field.

The poet lets us share in the joy she feels when her first child is born:

> When I hold you again in my arms, the blazing morning sun is rising up; it brightens our room and blesses you. The clustered red persimmons bend their branches with sparse, dry leaves at the back and the front yard. I can hear the daily activities of the morning: the train is rushing on the rails and whistling clamorously in the air; the neighbor's dogs bark resonantly; the morning cocks crow proudly as if announcing your birth to the world.

Her exquisite sensitivity to nature shines through this passage, when she tells of coming home from the hospital late on a winter night:

> The air is cutting and crispy; the sky is impeccably clear blue with shades of darkness; tiny flickering stars are on its farthest dome, and the white Milky Way sweeps as a long white trail. The white florescent full moon is hanging at the meridian in the vacant space and seems like a single giant universal street light lighting up the sleeping earth.

Finally, because she has the soul of a poet, Doctor Rhee is able to give words to her love for her profession. She delivers a baby, and she writes to her doctor daughter:

> Hyun A, don't we have the best profession? I will remember this moment always as one touched by a shaft of sacred light. All the labor, all the sacrifice, all the years of study seem to culminate in this one transcendent moment. For I am a doctor. I am here to help bring life into the world. And I will write about how this came to be.

And so this lovely little woman—wife, mother, medical doctor, writer, grandmother, citizen—passes her torch on to her daughter. That torch is contained in this beautiful, inspiring, humbling story—the autobiography of Doctor Chi Sun Rhee.

Elizabeth Ulrich Hoobler
Emeritus Professor of English,
Kent State University

Preface

Dear Hyun A,

Today in my den while rearranging cluttered books, the old and new, I discovered many notebooks of years long passed and stacks of papers piled in three-ring binders carefully labeled: five volumes of my poems, *Solitary Walking, Divine Journey Book One, Book Two,* four volumes called *Daily Thoughts,* book reviews, journals.... They were scattered everywhere in the room, distracting my eyes and mind, so many that I wanted to throw them all away to clean up the room, as I would have thrown away old patients' charts that were past term. And then I had a sudden idea: what if I filter off the less successful scribbles and gather the ones that seem valuable to make a book for you, a book which would be my gift of love. If I don't do this, I will go the grave with my unfinished works, all turning to dust together.

If you have this gift, you will not miss me after I have left you forever because you will have my words and my spirit. And I thought, you will then understand what it was to be a woman—wife, mother, medical doctor, writer, grandmother, citizen—in an era that is long gone and so better understand a woman's position and role in your own time and place. I can help you to know your heritage, gender, race, and perhaps the quirks of history. I cherish you, my daughter, my spirit, as one who will honor my gift.

I know now my time draws near to the end, for my eyes grow dimmer, all sound is fainter, my memory fails, my vigor wanes. It is time that I should hand the flame of my torch to you, the next and new generation.

Contents

—1—

To the New Land

Dear Hyun A,

Let me tell you how you came to be an American. It all began long ago.

Our adventure to the United States, the new promised land, demands a long journey away from our home and homeland. "Dooh, dooooh—" bawling whistles, and blowing smoke, the local train dashes out from behind the curved mountain toward the railroad station. It gradually slows and hisses white steam from its jowls. A stationmaster in a dark blue uniform and a cap with two red stripes stands welcoming the approaching train, waving the triangular red flag to signal the stop. The black iron caterpillar halts with a clamorous clank, and its echoing jolt ripples to its tail. When I hear that sound, its whole weight crushes upon my heart. The time has come. It is to me like fate, inevitable: we must go away from you to a foreign land thousands of miles away—and you and your two little brothers must stay here. Now there is no choice. We—your mom and dad—must separate from our three children. Of course we grieve for our relatives and friends, but they are adults. But you are eleven years old, Steve five, and Robert only two, and in his grandmother's arms.

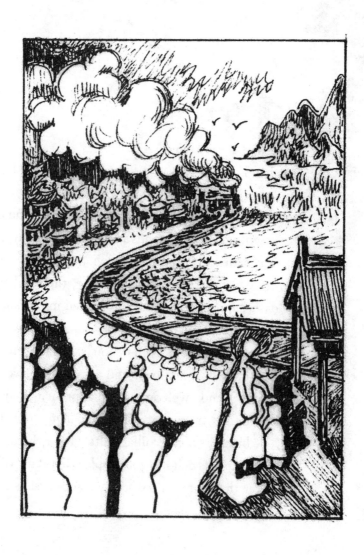

Around noon of June 22, 1969, a surge of people bounce on the concrete platform of Kwangju provincial station waiting for the train's arrival. They are your dad's and my families and relatives; professors and students from Chosun University where your dad worked as Chairman in the Department of Physics; doctors and nurses from the National Chonman Medical School where I trained and worked. A quiet mood pervades the air despite the swarms of crowds— blended expressions of sadness but at the same time, excitement. Our families feel special sorrow at losing us. Multiple rails flash; the heat of the searing sun shimmers on the lines of steel. People wipe sweat from their brows. Bystanders can see that an extraordinary event is occurring. Both sides of the families surround us to hold our hands to say good-bye, not knowing when they can expect our return. I hold Robert tightly to the last minute, but he is too young to realize what is happening. And your daddy and I hug your grandmother and aunts and great aunts and uncles and Steve and you, having no time to reach out to everyone. I embrace your grandmother again last of all. "Don't worry about your children," she says in a choked voice, "succeed in what you both want to be." Your dad and mom step up the stairs to the train. The black caterpillar starts its hissing engines, the white steam shrouds the wheels, the steam whistle cries "Dooh dooh dooooh," and it begins to depart from the Kwangju provincial station. I see the tears streaking Steve's cheeks under his white baseball cap as he holds his uncle's hand. You know more than he does, but you stand calm, wiping your tears as you watch your mom and dad go away from you. You are as beautiful as Cinderella dressed in her ball gown. I bought you the prettiest dress—a pink plum-flower-patterned white dress, with long lace ruffles at your sleeves and cascades of lace down the wide skirt. Your beauty tortures me.

The stationmaster's red flag waves to the driver of the train, and the crowd's white hands and white handkerchiefs are a sea of waving. We stand at the edge of the train step to see your figures until you are out of sight. We wave back and thank and thank again all the crowd's kindness and friendship. But tears blur my vision. I feel as if I am opening the door of death, leaving the three of you behind as though I never can see you again. What a dreadful experience to go through as the mother of three children! Beneath the waving I seem to hear the crowd whispering:

> They are out of their minds, they are all too crazy. Why in the world do they have to go, forsaking three little children and giving them to their old mother! They both have the highest achievements, professions that most people only dream of having: Sung Hi is Chairman of the Physics Department at Chosun University; Chi Sun is a board-certified obstetrician and gynecologist. It is hard to understand them. Most of all they are not young—mid forties. How can they survive in a foreign land with a foreign language among an alien race? The more we think of them, the more they appear as fools! Absolutely absurd!

The crowd's dismayed faces pass by before my blurring eyes and press my heavy heart. I feel I have just committed an enormous crime.

The train speeds on. I press my face to the window, and the more I think that this is the last time to see our homeland, the more I feel that everything I see is beautiful and significant. The ranges of endless mountains, rank on rank, the green pines, the plains wide or narrow—they symbolize our land and people who are ever strong, stately, and young like them. The rice plants of darkest green cover the expanse of the plains; in the distance a band of farmers in white—

wearing long pants rolled up to the knees and wide-brimmed straw hats—are working in the rice field. A group of women squat to follow the furrows of vegetation at the foot of the mountains to weed and to tend the vegetables and barley and cotton. Holding the reins, a straw-hatted man drives an oxcart loaded with cotton bales. It rolls heavily over the steep gravel road; behind it hurries a woman with a big bamboo basket loaded with lunch for the farmers. At the foot of the mountains, small thatches of farmhouses nestle on the red hills like gray mushrooms in wooded sunny nooks. A group of farmers sits and picnics in the shade. Here and there glimmering streams peep out of verdant rice fields. On the distant horizon, hazy blue air veils the dark mountain crests. The winding course of rivers in the plains supplies the water of life to all the plain as the big arteries of our bodies carry our blood. The sun has chased away all the clouds, and the sun reigns alone in the infinite sky. As the sun sinks beyond the western horizon, the black caterpillar arrives at the main train station at Seoul.

Why are we leaving our homeland? Your dad dreamed, as all men do. He had dreamed first of becoming an inventor like Thomas Edison or other immortals in the field of science, winning the Nobel Prize for his genius. However, by his mid forties, he was aware that he could not reach the level that he wanted to achieve. He felt he was too old for sharpening his brain for theories and devices. For this reason he shifted his interest and energy into quite a different channel, political science. He has always believed that political power and systems and leadership decide a nation's and a world's direction. He desired to use his ability for our nation's progress in politics, economics, science, and technology. Therefore, he decided to go abroad to a democratic country such as the United States to study and to learn how to help our own country develop.

My situation depended on your dad. In the summer of 1969 I obtained certification from the National Board of Obstetrics and Gynecology. Soon afterward, your dad threw a thunderbolt: would I like to follow him to the United States or would I prefer to stay home with our three children and practice medicine? Financially he had taken care of me, purchasing for me a private house to be used as a hospital. He was going to the United States to study political science and to acquire a Ph.D.; his decision to go abroad is unalterable. He said, "I promise I will come back home in triumph." I pondered for hours about the risks and benefits of leaving with him, and of staying at home with you children. I finally went to your grandmother to discuss leaving you children with her so that I might go with your dad. I said, "If I decide to go abroad, I don't want to risk the children's education and growth under an oppressive foreign culture and people. I want to go there first to see whether circumstances are fit to raise the children, as well as whether I myself can adjust to foreign medicine." I asked my mother to give me one year as a testing period. After one year, if all conditions were not met, I planned to come back home; if circumstances allowed us to bring the children with us, then we would send for the children. My mother graciously accepted the difficulty of caring for three little children.

Why did I decide to go with your dad, leaving you in Korea? First, even though your dad promised to come back home, I have seen what has happened to intellectuals and professors who go abroad to foreign countries, leaving their family behind. Some of them never come back. No one thought that these men—some even in your dad's department at the university—would ever forsake their wives and children. I didn't want to risk the chance of losing my husband. The second reason was this: if I could find the opportunity, I wanted to solve some of the frustrating enigmas in my own profession. In our medical schools we use Western textbooks, translating the English into the Korean language. But knowing the principles presented in those books and applying those principles is frustrating indeed: I don't have the proper tools to diagnose the diseases, no medicines to treat patients effectively, no proper materials, no advanced instruments for surgeries. I know all the materials, tools, medicines described in the textbooks are available in the United States. I wanted to go there and see how American medical doctors are applying those things in their practice.

These are the reasons for leaving you, my daughter—we hoped to bring you to a better world.

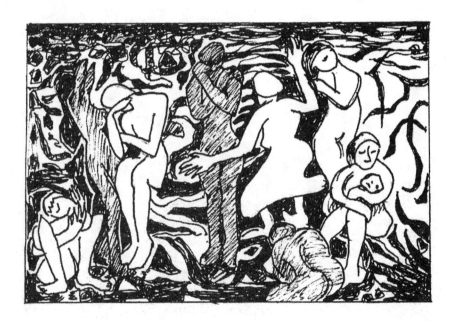

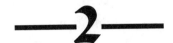

—2—

Arranging the Marriage

Dear Hyun A,

Who were these people who in middle age left their country behind? To understand them, you must understand something about the country they left behind.

Let me tell you about Korea in 1956, the year your mom and dad were married. It was a country divided, still bearing the scars of war, but we were beginning to recover. The times were changing suddenly—like the monsoon rains flooding the desert—and one of the greatest changes was in our traditions. I was at the forefront of those changes. You see, I was a professional woman. You see me now at twenty-three, and I have the job as a teacher at Kwangju Girls High School that I have always yearned for. But your grandmother worried about my aging without a husband. By Korean tradition, I am already a little old for marriage—girls usually marry between seventeen and twenty-two. And so one midsummer evening I expressed my decision your grandmother and your uncle: "I would like to marry and have children." I truly make them happy.

I had been thinking about marriage for a long time. By Korean tradition, there is no dating in junior high or high school; after reaching seven years of age, boys and girls are not permitted to sit together. But I had had one date; it lies deep in the recesses of my memory. It took place when I was twenty-one during the final year of Educational College.

As the springtime is the mating season for the feathers and fish, so the spring has an influence on men to seek their own partners. For the warm sun suddenly thaws out the frozen earth, the force of life emerging from the darkness of the soil bursts forth; the splendor of blossoms begins smiling everywhere from the gardens, yards, hills, and fields. In that season, unexpectedly, came my first date.

§   §   §

In 1953, Syung Man Kim is one of my classmates in Educational College, which focuses on training secondary school teachers who major in physics and mathematics. The college is affiliated with Chonmam University Medical School, and it does not have its own library. For this reason, the college students study at the Medical School Library together. Syung Man has a good brain and can solve difficult problems in all our subjects. He is ambitious to succeed in whatever he attempts to do. He seems intentionally to seek a quiet place to think and to read. He not only distinguishes himself in physics, but writes articles in the school periodical.

Four girl classmates—among the eighty in our class—study together with boy students, discussing the clues and answers to the

problems. One Saturday afternoon in the middle of the second-year
spring term, we are in the library where a few students are scattered
in that hollow, quiet room. I am in deep frustration, having come up
against a problem I cannot solve. Then I sense—without looking—
that somebody is standing at the right side of my desk. I look up to
see Syung Man; he smiles an abashedly gentle smile.

"Chi Sun, would you like to go out with me to the Seoul Tearoom?"

"When?"

"Now, any time that you are ready."

"Ooh, my head is just about to explode! You are my rescuer!"

"Really? I am glad to hear that!" he says, widening his quiet eyes,
and he almost touches his hands together to clap.

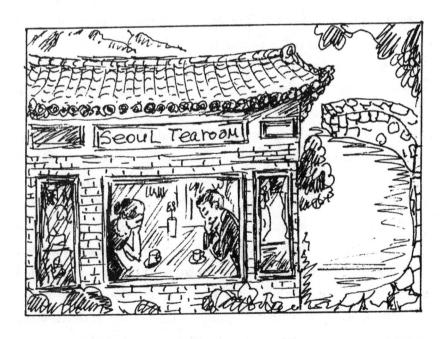

In the Seoul Tearoom the elite of society sit and are conversing.
The strains of a classic waltz sound softly through the pleasant, small,

low-ceilinged room. Pictures brushed with black Chinese ink—irises
on the rocks, snowy peaks, and rivers with boats—and scrolls with
black brush letters of axioms hang on the beige walls. Gold and silver fish are swimming through the green seaweed in the long basin
on the receiving counter. Their long-spread white fins and tails are
fanning the water. The waitress brings two flower-decorated cups of
Sang Whwa tea. The tea is thick, pitch black, with small white pinenuts
and red pieces of sliced dates floating on the surface. The wispy, delicious steam curls up. The hot tea needs time to cool.

"Is your head flame extinguished now?" Syung Man shows his
concern.

"Much better, but not completely yet. Soon it will be all right."

Though we stare at our own steaming cups in silence for a while,
I can see his complaisant countenance, which glows with light-
heartedness. And he wipes his broad face with two open palms as if
to wash his face and mops round his mouth with his left palm. His
right elbow is on the table, and his right palm buttresses his chin.
Hesitatingly, yet in a very sweet tone, he asks me, "What are you
going to do in the future?" and he rivets his eyes upon my eyes; the
intensity of his gaze melts my soul. We had never had this sort of
private question before.

"I would like to teach in Kwangju City, since our house and
relatives live here."

"How many brothers and sisters do you have?"

"I have one brother and three sisters. My brother graduated from
Seoul National University with a chemistry major. He was awarded
the President's prize at the commencement ceremony."

"Oh, then he must be distinguished in school records; he must
have had the highest score among Seoul National University graduates," he says.

"Yes, he did! I am very proud of him. I believe he will discover or invent something great in the future. What do you want to be in the future?" I start drinking the tea; he follows.

"I have changed my mind," he says. "I am not going to be a teacher after graduating from this college next year. I will continue my study of physics at Seoul National University, and then I will go to the United States for the advanced study of nuclear physics."

"It will be an awfully hard and long way for you."

"I know that! But there is no great future for me if I stay in a secondary school teaching job," he says. His sharp chin and drawn mouth exhibit his determination. His piercing eyes are fixed on my eyes continuously. He asks if I want another cup of tea. Then Syung Man asks me again, "What are you going to do this afternoon? If you don't have any special engagement, I would like to spend this afternoon with you so we can go walking in the park." His body is firm but his voice and its tone sound pleading.

But I must debate with myself. I don't hesitate to accept his offer because he is an excellent student, competing with me in every subject: physics, mathematics, chemistry. Besides his academic achievement, he is physically fit and personally attractive, having a quiet yet brave character. My only reluctance to go with him is fear of the contemptuous eyes and malignant rumors of the public— friends, professors, family. I don't want to be a despised object. I stare at my empty cup in silence. I brood over it: now, I am twenty-one, an adult. I can decide whether behavior is proper or not. I decide to go with him—I know well who he is—to spend one afternoon, which may be a good break and experience for me.

We climb a long flight of steps to the watch stand at the Sa Gik Park and look over the thickly packed Kwangju City encompassed by faraway mountain ranges, hazy and blue-black. We move on to the park's hilltop where the towering red pines grow together, offering shelter and a playground for the birds. The dead needles of pines are spread over the acres and acres of ground beneath them. The large black cones fall, lying like black birds perched on the red carpet. The white streams of pine resin stain the red trunks, sending forth a clean pungent scent all over the hill. As we go down to the back side of the park, the wafery tender leaves on the ancient maples are fluttering silver in a breath of wind. Beside them, Syung Man and I sit on the turf and look down on the dark-green pine forests under the warm sun. A pair of ravens are crying and flying over the trees. Syung Man sits closer to me, and he takes my hand. At this moment, his hand is like an electric shock plate. The unexpected act halts my blood's circulation and then lets it flow counter currently; my mind is paralyzed by his galvanized electric hand over my hand so that I am unable to shake my hand free from his. He repeats and emphasizes his future plans to be a great physicist as if he wants me to have sure confidence in him. He again draws his conversation to his dream: "Once I seriously took literature into consideration, but my natural endowments for physics will be more fruitful than writing."

An hour passes by; he asks me if I could possibly go to see the movie *Syngohara* with him. "Oh, yes," I reply promptly. "I hear the movie is good, so I had already planned to go." I see him smiling contentedly.

When we enter the huge theater, the seats are almost filled. On the stage, a gigantic purple curtain is drawn closed. Inside, the room is dark with very dim lights. The movie is so dramatic that I remember it still. It is a tragic love story between the prince of a small kingdom and a gypsy girl who is the daughter of a gypsy chieftain. Several hundred members of a gypsy group settle in the valley at the base of the mountains. A feudal lord lives in a castle on one of the mountains. He has a young son who suffers from somnambulism. One night at the full moon he walks from his castle to the fields while he is sleeping; he sees a beautiful girl at the stream and walks toward her. The most beautiful girl among all the gypsy girls, enticed by the blue moonlight, sits alone by the mirror of the water and listens to the murmurs of the silvery foam. Suddenly she sees a man's black image in the water. She is frightened to have a young man standing beside her, but his attire and good-looking figure and stately air show that he is a prince.

The prince and the gypsy fall in love and meet every night. But gypsies are wanderers, and the time comes to move to another territory. Syngohara, the gypsy girl, realizes she is pregnant, and she is desperate to stay with the prince. She pretends to her people to have the plague, and they leave her on the spot and fly away from her. She and the prince and the baby live in the castle. But the gypsy horde comes again in their season, and they discover Syngohara is alive and living with the prince. Gypsy mobs attack the castle and fight with the warriors of the castle to get her back. Almost everyone in the castle—Syngohara, the prince, and the baby prince—dies from the gypsies' swords and arrows. Even though the castle is flooded with blood, their immortal love triumphs over their mortal death.

While watching the movie, Syung Man holds my hand. Sometimes with his other hand he rubs my hand that is in his palm. The love of Syngohara and the prince transfers to us, making us feel closer; as the hours pass, his hand makes me feel that his skin becomes a part of my own.

When the movie is over and we scramble through the crowd at the theater's doorway, the red sun is setting above the gray horizon; dark, thin strips come over the right center of the dying sun and split it into two semicircles above and below. The dark mass of clouds above the sun dazzles in a gold burst; the rest of the sky is all white. The trees stand motionlessly on either side of the street as if they are in deep slumber. Nonetheless, the crowd on the street walks briskly, rustling the air. Syung Man escorts me home with a quiet, happy glow like the setting sun. This first date suddenly awakens me to realize that it is time to seek my life partner and to have my own family.

§   §   §

At age twenty-three, I go to my family and say that I am ready to be married. Conventionally, professional matchmakers, either men or women, play a great role in the success of a marriage, but the role of matchmaker can be taken by parents, friends, or relatives. Your grandmother calls matchmakers well known to our family and tells them, "I want to give my daughter in marriage."

Matchmakers know well which family is suitable to which family; in the Korean culture, a family's name, status, and ranking are primary conditions when arranging a marriage. Our matchmakers bring my mother information from various houses that seem strong candidates for a successful marriage. From this information our family sorts out four candidates for me. The first is a twenty-five-year-old banker; the first son of Mr. Kim, the president of one of the provincial banks. The second is thirty-four, a university professor in the chemistry department and the second son of Mr. Choi, the president of a textile manufacturing company. The third is a surgeon of twenty-nine and the second son of the surgeon Dr. Shin. And the fourth, also twenty-nine, is Professor Rhee of the university physics department and the third son of Mr. Rhee, a businessman who passed away some years ago.

Even though the older members of our family are most interested in the men's families. I am more concerned with the person than with his name. After all, I am the one who will live with that man, not my family. Hyun A, I am in different circumstances when compared to most women of my age. At this time in Korea, only a handful of women have professional careers. And even these, once they marry, usually stay at home and become housewives. I have a different idea because I feel called to a shining greatness. My new ideas cause our family complications and delay in making a final decision.

Before I choose a husband, the following conditions are to be met. First, I never want my career to be encumbered by marriage. This condition is of great consequence to me. Hyun A, I do not wish to marry someone who is the first son of his family. In our Korean social system, the first son is responsible for his parents and all his siblings; moreover, he is the only heir to the family wealth. I would automatically be bound by an unseen yoke of the system; consequently, my progress would be stalled. I would be a slave of convention and unable to take advantage of the new opportunities in society. Hyun A, you will ask me, "Why do you need freedom so much?" Because without my freedom, I won't know my own potential. Without freedom, an individual can never discover or develop his potential. Second, it is an essential condition that I find a man who not only has success in his own career but also understands my status and supports me. He must be willing to grow with me independently and individually, both of us pursuing our own fields. Hyun A, how can I take care of a large family—both care for his parents and also educate all of his brothers and sisters and care for them until they marry? Not that I want to escape from my duty—if I should become only a housewife, that would be my job and I would not look outside that job. But I want both a home and a career, and I can only have both with the right man.

By our custom, if both families are interested in interviewing (*Seun*) each other, the matchmakers arrange the date. The woman's male relatives—father or uncles or brothers—go to the man's house and interview the prospective bridegroom. The family may offer a savory lunch or a sumptuous dinner. Conversely, from the man's side, women—the mother, aunts, daughters-in-law—go to the woman's family and interview the prospective bride. The interviewers report their impressions to their daughter or son: the person's appearance, bearing, personality, interests.... If their daughter and son are eager to meet each other, their parents allow the children to see each other before making a final decision.

Your uncle and great uncle make their visits; they give me their impression of the banker, Mr. Kim. He has a good family and family name in society; he is a tall, good-looking, pleasant, ambitious, and promising young man. They think if I marry him, my happiness can be assured. They also tell me about Professor Choi: he is thin, with a pale complexion, handsome, and quiet. He does give them an indifferent impression in other things besides his profession. In particular, he looks old, having a large area of frontal baldness. They think if I marry him, he will look more like a father to me than a husband. And their impression of Dr. Shin is this: he has a medium-stout frame and well-formed features. His father has a good name, and he himself is popular with his patients. Your uncle and great-uncle like his sociable personality. They are excited about both Mr. Kim and Dr. Shin. Finally, they are impressed by the family of Professor Rhee— that family is nationally linked to the government and Congress, and is locally linked to the provincial official positions—but they are not impressed by the person himself. Professor Rhee is healthy and handsome, but his manners are unacceptable. When they interviewed him, he stayed just five minutes. "I must leave," he said. "I have a class to teach." Then, without even smiling, he hurried away. Worse, they hear rumors about him: he is an abnormal person; he does not hang around with his friends; he does not go to church. He studies all the time. Sometimes he stays to study at the physics laboratory until one, two, or three o'clock in the morning; sometimes he even sleeps at the lab. When he graduated from the university, even though he was receiving top honors, he didn't attend the commencement ceremony and instead studied all evening. Your uncle and great uncle adamantly object to my marrying him.

Meanwhile, Dr. Shin requests to meet me directly at the Boo Rae Ock, the custard and tea house. With my mother's permission, I go to meet him. He is very enthusiastic about seeing me and seems eager to marry and have a family. He is very considerate and kind, saying, "If you marry me, you won't have to work at the school. You won't have to worry about money, you can have anything you want. You can just stay home and take care of me and the children."

He asks me if I want something special and orders many delicious cakes, tea, and ice cream. After the interview is over, he takes me home in a taxi. It is a very moving moment. I like him because he is healthy, can express his feelings clearly, and has a warm, passionate personality. I have a tug-of-war in my own mind.

And then Professor Rhee's matchmaker comes to our matchmaker. Professor Rhee wants to see me person to person at the Boo Rae Ock tea room. This tea and cake house is cozy and private; it has good snacks and is the best place to socialize. The popsicle machine makes a little constant noise in the background. Professor Rhee is sitting in a booth waiting for me. He asks me what I want. "I like to drink milk," he says, "and the French prime minister likes to drink milk too." I cannot answer him right away. He orders two glasses of milk and says, "Try it!" and he slides the glass toward me. He asks me what I want to do with my life—after marrying, how will I continue my career? I do not reply directly to his many questions. I want him to bring out what interests him about me. He does not try to please me with delicious foods as did Dr. Shin. He doesn't seem to care about my comfort at home after marriage; instead his tone implies that he would want me to strive for my own fulfillment in my profession. "I have heard," he says, "that you are good at your teaching and like to study."

He orders two cups of Korean Ginseng tea and two pieces of custard. "Right now I am teaching my students the Quantum Theory," he says. "Next spring quarter, I will teach Physics of Hydrodynamics." He says that the courses are interesting but entail lots of time to prepare. He does not linger with me; he does not call a taxi—we go home our separate ways. It is the middle of December; the entire sky is gray; blowing winds' wings freeze in the air. And the remnants of snow mixed with the street mud are piled at the sidewalks as though salt mounds lie at the salt sea.

That night I toss about in my bed till the night stillness deepens because of Professor Rhee's intense, large black eyes, his rolling crystal voice, and his focused interest. Obviously his manner and bearing are unique, strong, and overpowering. He never uttered a word about what he would like me to do if I should marry him. I think about the information I've learned about him from my family and from other people; I try to understand why people say that he is abnormal, that he has something missing, that he is immature, an imbecile in social affairs. The more I analyze his characteristics, the more I feel him rising above the people who gossip about him. He is levitated in the high air as an extraordinary shining genius.

Hyun A, how do I come to such elevation? Think! I ask, does he smoke? Does he drink? Did he flunk? Did he have money from his parents to go to school like an ordinary student? Did he blaspheme God's name? And an answer comes to me,

> He does not smoke. He does not drink. He is always at the
> top of any of his classes. He paid all of his school expenses
> himself without any help from his older brother. And above
> all, he believes in God.

People condemn him as immature because he does not hang around with them. Hyun A, if he is with them, he is an ordinary man like them. But how can he be the best in his field if he does all the things that ordinary people do? Most of all he has to make his own living: during the day he goes to school, and at night he teaches high school students, a moonlighting job that allows him to support himself. After thinking this through, I am convinced that he is a fine man, far above all the people who deride him. Best of all, he is the third son of Mr. Rhee senior. This condition gives me the chance to develop my own potential. I decide that he is the best candidate for me to marry.

Now more and more my family is pressing me to marry either the banker Mr. Kim or Dr. Shin. Mr. Kim is a good candidate but not for me, since he is the first son of seven siblings. Dr. Shin is also an excellent candidate, but he is not fit for my life because he wants me to abandon my career. I ask my family to tell these men that I am no longer considering them as marriage candidates. And I announce to my family that I want to marry Professor Rhee. My determination causes rage and conflict. They are stunned at what I say. But I stand up for my conviction: "He is a genius and a great man. I like him for the very points that you hold against him. Those are the points that make him great. For those I want to marry him. I will take the consequences."

My mother, my brother, and my uncle exhort me again and again to think more carefully and to change my mind. They paint the picture of my misery, living with this abnormal man. They beg me to give up Professor Rhee and to consider the other two candidates before they change their minds about me. I am afraid to come home from school because I can hardly bear hearing my family's bitter criticism of my stupid decision to throw my fortune away. But eventually they give in and reluctantly agree to allow me to marry Professor Rhee.

Then our matchmakers arrange to send the written marriage contract form (*Sa Sung*) first to my family and then to Professor Rhee's. My family signs the form and sends it on; however, Rhee's family is silent for more than two weeks. As a result, our family thinks the Rhees are no longer interested in me. I feel defeated in the battle-field of marriage; I realize that to marry is not simple or even happy but becomes a confusing quandary. However in a sense my family is happy. The other two candidates are still eager to marry me.

One day when I come home from school, I see my matchmaker waiting for me. She says, "I will explain what happened during the last three weeks at the Rhees'":

> Before seeing you, Professor Rhee and his uncle interviewed a maiden at the town of Soon Chun. She is a girl of twenty-three, an elementary school teacher. Her beauty, and the Kim name and fortune, are celebrated in the town. Her family received their visitors with a feast, and they strongly impressed Professor Rhee's uncle. But the professor is interested only in you. So his uncle and he had a furious dispute. The uncle called his nephew an imbecile. "You don't know," he said, "anything about society! What have you been learning at school?" He was so angry that he didn't speak to his nephew for three weeks. Nevertheless, Professor Rhee never gave in. Finally, yesterday his uncle surrendered to him. That's the reason that I am here now.

People don't know how warm and good is the heart of Professor Rhee. They don't know his genius.

In two days, the Rhees send us the written form of the marriage contract with its brushed black-ink writing in Chinese characters. After receiving this, my brother sends our written agreement to the Rhees. Whether I have chosen the right man or the wrong man, I have crossed the Rubicon.

Once the written marriage agreement is exchanged, your grandmother calls a professional fortuneteller to our house and lets her pick an auspicious day for our marriage. The fortuneteller can be a man or a woman, but women are predominant. Our fortuneteller sits cross-legged on the floor near the center of the east wall of the room, unfolds her black portable desk, and places upon it a worn, magenta-covered book. She closes her eyes, holding her hands together on her lap, and rocks her body from side to side for a few minutes as if invoking the aid of divine power. She asks your grandmother, "What is your daughter's birthday? Give me the year, month, day, and specific hour." She still swings her body with her eyes closed. When your grandmother replies, she counts silently, putting each finger from the index to the little finger against her thumb. Then she opens her eyes and fingers through the book, which is written with Chinese characters and has colorful illustrations. Within the book, everyone's fate is predestined and pictured in color by the four pillars of his birth—year, month, date, and hour. She calculates something with fingers and lips as before and leafs through the book again and again.

Finally she looks up. "Ah, indeed it is splendid!" she exclaims. "A splendid day!" Her pale face glows with joy, and she claps her right thigh with her tiny hand. "I have never seen four pillars of such good fortune!" She clicks her tongue a few times and says once more, "Astonishing!" Fingering the pictures of her book, she cries, "Madam Yoo, look, look here! These golden sheaves are stacked in mounds by the magnificent mansion. Ah! So many children in the house, too. In front of the house, the golden waves of rice fields extend to the horizon. Madam! The propitious day is May second, 1956."

One day Professor Rhee calls me and asks me to go out to see a movie at the Kwangju Theater. This time his appearance is remarkably changed: he is cheery; he wears better clothes; he is softer, kinder, and more talkative. He shows genuine affection to me. "I like to see movies," he says. "Do you like movies?" He makes me forget everything just to respond to him with joy.

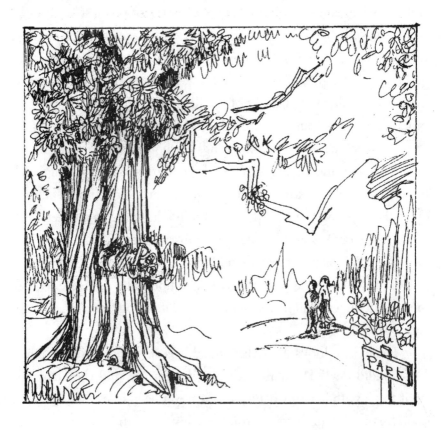

Only two theaters are available in the big city. The seats are long wooden benches. He leads me to the third center row from the rear. The movie is about Marilyn Monroe, who is singing, plucking her guitar, and crossing a river in some area of the American West. I do not know exactly what is happening in the story. My attention is not on the movie but on my surging happiness and his affable glowing.

When we get out of the dark theater, he takes me to that Boo Rae Ock for tea, Sang Wha Cha, in which small white pinenuts are floating in the thick black ginseng liquid; a wisp of curling steam smelling of herbs rises from our tea cups. It soothes our tense affections. When we are ready to go home, he takes two notebooks and hands one to me. "This is for you," he says, "this is for me. I want you to keep a diary now. I will do the same." What an extraordinary man! How many engaged women can expect to receive a blank notebook to let her write her daily thoughts?

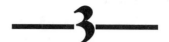

The Wedding

Dear Hyun A,

Your mom and dad were late in marrying—
he was thirty, I twenty-three. According to Korean standards, our marriage was exceptionally
late. For example, your dad's younger brother and
sister were already married and had children. Your
father's parents had married at seventeen; your
mother's father married at seventeen, and his wife
was sixteen! Your dad explained that he married
late because he wanted to be a preeminent physicist like one of the Nobel Prize winners, and marriage would get in his way.

In our time the drive for simplification of the
traditional Korean wedding ceremony began; the
Korean government encouraged that simplification. Today the wedding often takes place at the
church or at a professional wedding hall and is
conducted by a pastor or a priest. The western

rituals result in real savings in both time and money. But in our time some conventional families stubbornly clung to their traditions. Both your our families valued their own customs and held their children's nuptials according to the traditions of thousands of years of culture. Let me tell you about our wedding.

The weather is very important to the wedding day. Superstition says it predicts the happiness of the marriage. In Korea, a brief shower in summer is rare. Once it rains, it stays raining for days. Hyun A, my memory nudges me to tell you about the rain on the day and night before our wedding day. How it tormented me!

The ceaseless rain seems to curse our wedding. By midnight I am far more anxious about the weather than about the wedding itself. My thousand unspoken prayers are not answered. I lie in my bed and I can hear the pouring rain beat down upon the tiles on the roof as though splitting them to pieces; its drops cut splashes on the watery ground; its stream mutters down through the gutters. What if the guests do not show up at our wedding? Our ceremony will be held under a tent pitched in the front yard. There is no alternative— there are too many guests to fit in my home's ceremonial hall.

I imagine the worst: the bridegroom and bride and all the guests alike are soaked in the rain; the floors and kitchens are awash in mud; the crowds leave right after the ceremony without having a good time at the reception banquet or tasting our best foods and wines. The foods will spoil in the warm weather (at that time in the entire nation there were no refrigerators). My splitting head aches with the muddle. I am exhausted and fall into a sound sleep. Then suddenly I start astonished from my slumber, for everything is strangely silent. I open the door and look out of the room. It is a miracle! No more rain pours down; instead, the first blushing streaks of day dawn brightly under the fair sapphire sky with its blinking morning stars. Truly the curse of the rain is transformed into our blessing.

By custom the wedding ceremony must be held at the bride's home. The bride's parents are responsible for all expenses. Your grandfather, my father, had passed away; therefore your uncle—the first-born son—had become head of the family. He acted as my father and paid for everything.

The focus for the Korean wedding is the Korean wedding table set in the center of the tent pitched in the bride's yard. Everything on the table, and every ritual in the nuptials, is a symbol for the bridegroom and bride—for their union, ties, prosperity, chastity, and long, happy life. At noon, as the dazzling sun beams down, the guests fill our yard and elbow their way to the tent.

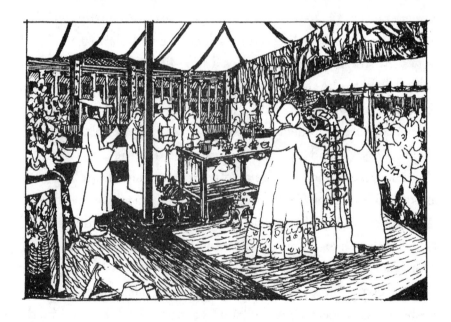

Within the white tent on the center of the ground is a large rectangular mahogany table. A live snow-white rooster with bloody red cockscombs and round glassy eyes is placed at the corner where the bridegroom will stand, and a brown-red-black hen is placed on the bride's side opposite the cock. A wooden carved duck and drake are put on the other two corners. These birds represent changeless life mates. Two bunches of straight, small bamboo trees, symbols of changelessness and honesty, are placed on each side at the center edge. These are connected to each other at the top by a braided red and blue thread that means that both persons are now united as one. Beside the bamboo are bundles of white and pink and purple paper flowers, fully blown like our national flower, the rose of Sharon, the Chinese rose. In the empty spaces of the table are piled all kinds of fruits on wide mahogany lacquered dishes—layers of apples, pears, dried dates, dried persimmons, peeled chestnuts, oranges; all kinds of sweets—beige malt candies, palm-sized-wide sweet rice wafers dredged with malt sweets and crumbles of popped rice *(Sanja)*, fried sweet crackers *(Yakguwa)*, steamed rice cakes layered with red beans *(Syru Dyuk)*—all of these typify sweet love and life that will stick together. A long noodle indicates a long life. At the center of the table, close to the dignitary conducting the ceremony, is a copper kettle with two small copper cups.

The Korean bridegroom wears a suit with its vest *(Gyugori, Bagy, Chocki)* and the wedding gown with the crown *(Samo Kwandae)*. Your daddy wears a light blue suit and a thick blue vest; his crown is of black hard net with three long horns jutting from the top center and both sides. The long black wedding gown falls to his feet. On his chest is a large square emblem embroidered with two flying storks in a sky with a red sun; red pine trees are beneath them. The emblem connotes an ever-young, free, happy life mate. The emblem is connected to a stiff steel-segmented belt covered by the same black cloth; on each segment golden characters are engraved that symbolize many children, wealth, happiness, long life, and health. Your daddy wears mid-shin-high black boots and looks just like the King of the Rhee Dynasty in the picture in our textbook. I am not supposed to look at anyone, particularly the groom. But I furtively glance at him. He makes me swell with pride. I have a hard time suppressing my joy.

I, the bride, wear a traditional costume: a long-sleeved blouse and long trailing skirt in jade green, a pair of white fabric socks that reach to my shin, and jade rubber shoes shaped like boats. Over the blouse I wear a long, pale green wedding gown with long rectangular sleeves from which hang twenty-inch strips of cloth of crimson, primrose, snow, sapphire, turquoise, and rose; the crimson strings tie at the front. On my head is a black satin crown embroidered with colorful beads and dangling long-chained pearls. At the back of my head is a golden hairpin eight inches long, etched at one side with an elaborate flower. (I do not recall how my maids worked with my short hair so that pin stayed on. But I do remember that long bright ribbons hung from it that reached to the hips and swung down to the thighs as I bowed down.)

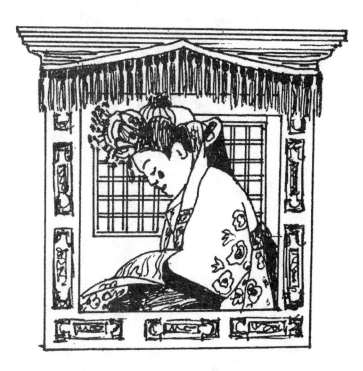

What do I do with my hands during this ceremony? About three yards of white silk cloth cover my hands and drape over them; I must hold my two hands together, never letting go. My eyes are cast down all through the ceremony and my mouth is closed tightly; I stand like a stone statue. Two maids hold my arms to help me do the many bows.

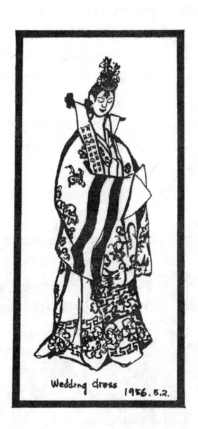

Wedding dress 1956. 5.2.

Our conductor is our relative; we call him Uncle Song Chon. He empties wine into one copper cup and carries it along the braided blue-and-red thread to the bridegroom, who drinks half of it. He then gives the cup with the rest of the wine to the bridesmaid, who brings the cup to the bride's lips and touches them, pretending to let the bride drink, and then gives it back to the conductor. Then the bride and groom bow to each other many times—I can't remember how many times. Now the bridegroom's and the bride's spirit flow together, are exchanged, and are united into one. The uncle announces the marriage to all the guests. The men and women guests separate from one another and go into the house for the reception banquet.

After the feasting of the bridal reception, it is close to twilight. Your daddy's friends fill the largest room in our house; they put the bridegroom at the center of the eastern wall and begin their play, the so-called "dalliance." Now the friends become ruthless tyrants; the bridegroom becomes their blind slave who has no right to resist them. They command him to bring his bride and let her sit behind him. If he refuses, they beat his the soles of his feet with small hardwood clubs. They play all sorts of naughty tricks: they force him to feed his bride, to make her sing alone, and to sing a duet with her. In order to evade the blows, we sing our folk song "Arirang Ridge." One of my husband's friends tears off the long cloth tape that closes the top of his garment. The friends are glad that they have a new chance to torment him. This time he has to beg his wife to sew his torn tape. He tries to defy their order, but the more he stands up to them, the harder they beat him. I can see that his body is torn with his friends' brawls and blows. I rescue the poor bridegroom, forgetting to be shy. Otherwise the bones of his feet will break and be crushed. In the scuffle one of his socks slips off his foot; they force him to beg his bride, "Please put my sock on my foot!"

"Do your own thing," I say to him, "for yourself!"

No sooner do I say this than they all hush at once, as though the bride has committed blasphemy against man's supremacy. They never expected defiance against a man from a woman, particularly from a bride's mouth. Nonetheless, the outspoken cry spears their blind, traditional hearts. They may think their friend, the bridegroom, will suffer with a domineering wife; they will tease me always with that phrase: "Do your own thing."

And that is what your daddy helped me to do—"my own thing"—all the rest of my life.

§   §   §

Shortly past midnight, the end of the torturous dalliance closes the long day of the wedding. Now the night of the consummation of marriage has commenced beneath the heavens: blessings of the myriad stars in the Milky Way shower down upon us; the silent choir of the heavenly cherubs fills the fairest dark-blue sky.

According to our five-thousand-year tradition, the just-married couple spends the wedding night at the bride's home. For this reason the corner room in our house has been prepared for your daddy and me. Our white Korean paper made from mulberry fiber covers the open grids of the wooden doors. The fresh scent floats around all over the room.

A huge four-fold screen sits unfolded by the rear door and that side wall. Each fold is framed with dark, varnished wood. Inside the wood is a narrow border formed by five layers of different shades of red fabric. Inside the border, on a backdrop of white fabric, are embroidered traditional scenes that feature the happiness of marriage. Each fold of the screen has a different scene: two snow-white cranes flying in the night of the full moon, skimming over the pine trees that are evergreen all seasons round; a couple of proud peacocks, the male spreading out his splendid tail like a dazzling fan; a pair of birds resting on trees that bloom with enchanting flowers: roses of Sharon, pink China roses, and snow-pink blossoms on the plum trees in the spring snow; unbending evergreen bamboo; domineering mountain ranges and the unbroken flow of the rivers—all these are embroidered with colorful silk by women's hands.

New bedding made of silks and satins with luxuriant patterns of an over quilt *(Yible),* a mattress *(Yo),* cushions, and sheets—your grandmother made these with her own hands—are piled at one corner of the room. The mattress is already spread out at the place to make our bed. Two pillows lie neatly abreast at the mattress' edge. The pillow that is for your daddy is a long, soft column. On both edges are hard square boards. Either side of the hard board is shrouded over with embroidered flowers and feathers. I have round boards instead of square ones. Along both sides, the hems of the white pillowcases are ornamented with beautiful stitching.

When I cross the threshold, your daddy sits on the mattress to receive me. My two bridesmaids have dressed me in the gown and crown worn at the wedding ceremony during the daytime. They lightly hold each of my elbows and open the door and take me before him, handing me into his arms. Bowing to your daddy mutely, they retire from our room and close the door. Your daddy lets me sit beside him. Following the custom, he must now do the uncrowning and undressing of the bride. The bride must be silent and keep her eyes cast down, bending her head slightly forward, and await his movement. Your daddy wears his shirt (*Gyugori*) with its vest *(Chocki)* and trousers (*Bagy*), and white fabric socks tucked into both ends of the Bagy and tied with pale purple ribbons (*Denym*). He does not say a word and just sits by me straight and cross-legged. I can't imagine what his expression can be.

At the moment my two bridesmaids close our door, my fear grows and prevails over my happiness. I am young and naive, and now I am facing reality. I know very little about this man, but the nuptial tie has been accomplished. I am no longer free; I am responsible for another person besides myself. What will happen to me? I do not know. I feel lost, groping on the inevitable dark road. Where should I turn? My husband's silence prompts my heart's thumping faster and faster against my ribcage. I am trembling as I rock to and fro, and my hands become clammy and wet. Can he not see my misery? He comes closer to me. "Don't be afraid," he says. "I am your husband." And then he starts to follow his instinct and custom—probably he is more scared than I. After removing all of my ceremonial clothing, he reaches his big hand to the light bulb to turn it off. I feel that my crazily running heart has just stalled.

On the next day, the bright sunbeams shine through the white papered door to illuminate our room. We notice multiple finger holes poked through the door papers, both the door at the front and the door at the rear.

—4—

A New Life

Dear Hyun A,

Everywhere I look, the early summer sun—after the long rain—lights and warms every living thing on the fields and mountains; they are growing in green and becoming greener and greener every day, clothing the bare earth. Even though our wedding is over, my family continues to be busy during my last three days at home, receiving unending guests and preparing my departure to your daddy's home at Manghori, Yung Am County. By tradition, the bride has to bring gifts to the bridegroom's family. My family has to pack, to wrap, and to organize all the gifts to send to your daddy's family.

My apprehension escalates as the day to depart from my home draws near. I do not know your daddy's family. I have never been to Yung Am but have only heard the county's name. I am not going there for a trip or just to visit, but for a lifetime, becoming a part of your daddy's family. I am nervous because your daddy's family is well known for holding fast to orthodox traditions inherited from the aristocratic class. My background is different: since I turned twelve I have boarded at school away from home, plunged into the new era and exposed to the new open culture coming to Korea—unceremonious, pragmatic. But I don't want to give your daddy's family the impression that I am ignorant of our traditions (although some of them are indeed unreasonable, wasteful and slavish). Your daddy is a blazing star, not only to his family, but in all his village. He is the second professor in his family—his older brother became the first professor in Chosun University, but he died young. Now your daddy is the only professor in his entire village. I must show them that I deserve to be his counterpart. Under my mother's, aunts', and matchmaker's guidance, I have practiced the traditional ceremonial bow and regular formal bow countless times. I have been advised on how to use proper language as well as the titles and rankings of family and relatives, and how to behave in different rituals and replies. I feel as if I am a wild horse, captured, fenced, bridled.

By tradition, in three days a bride must leave her own home forever for her husband's home and then utterly belong to her husband's family. Once a woman marries a man, she has nothing to do with her own blooded family. That means she has to take care for her own new family as well as her husband's family. She is not responsible for her own blooded family. That will be the responsibility of her brothers, especially the oldest brother, who is responsible for his grandparents, parents, brothers and sisters; for the oldest son inherits all of his parents' property.

When the bride leaves her home, she has many many things to bring—not only gifts to every member of her husband's direct family but also to close relatives. But these gifts are a small portion compared to her own portion. Traditionally the bride's parents have to buy many necessities, including her and her husband's clothing for all four seasons, bureaus, dining tables, clothes chests, bedspreads, mattresses, pillows, cushions.... In order to do this, the bride's parents—besides overspending on their daughter's wedding—cannot help but be saddled with debt. For this reason, they say that if someone has three daughters or more, those daughters will take away the props and stays of her parents' home. Your daddy and I request your grandma and uncle not to prepare anything for us except gifts for your daddy's family.

At last, on the third morning after our wedding, the truck comes, and a few men including the driver load it with the mountainous presents. Now, you will ask me, "What kind of presents were they?" Chiefly clothes chests, quilts and mattresses, pillows and cushions made of silks and satins. For your daddy's grandmother and mother, there are classic dresses, blouses, and long skirts, three layers of separate underwear and fabric socks, and rolls of colorful silks and satins. There are dresses for all the families, including all of their children. Your daddy has a large family: three brothers and sisters. His uncle has a large family too—his great uncle's family, his two aunts' families—they all must have gifts. We bring food—not just a few boxes but countless large or small bamboo boxes of sweets such as wheat gluten, fried sweet rice cakes, a variety of candies and cakes, many different types of regular rice or sweet rice cakes, fish, cooked beef and pork, fruits of oranges, pears, apples, dried persimmons, dried dates, ginkgo nuts, chestnuts....

The heavy-laden truck drones away from our home and turns the corner of the street; next, the sleek dark taxi carrying the newly-wedded couple, the bridegroom's uncle, and the matchmaker follows the path of the truck. Your daddy and I turn back and wave through the taxi's back window to the weeping family.

It is about one hundred miles from Kwangju to Yung Am. Even as the taxi slips out from the city, the gravel road is wide and well developed. The rough gravel has been ground to sand by thousands of continually rolling wheels. The road is smooth, without much jolting and jerking as it winds over the rivers, on the plains, and around the mountains. Unbroken as the landscape is, I seem to be blind. I can't see the landscape; instead the voices of your grandmother and great aunts and matchmakers are ringing and whirling in my ears:

> Put your hands crossed over your brow; don't talk loudly or very much; reply with engaging smiles rather than sounds; don't eat too much or too fast; move slowly, gently, and gracefully; use respectful words to elders; don't stand straight before elders but always keep your head slightly down; as soon as you wake up, put on your make-up and dress formally; don't flirt with your husband before others....

All of these directions blend into a chaotic mass, blinding my vision. Midway through the trip, your daddy puts his left arm about my shoulders. At that instant, your daddy's uncle turns his head back, giving a menacing look to your daddy, who at once withdraws his outstretched arm. No one has spoken a word throughout the drive but your great uncle. He alone can talk if he wants to.

When the taxi arrives at Yung Am Town, it is greeted by two formally dressed maids and four costumed paraquin bearers. The men wear black caps without brims; from atop the cap a long black thong with white fluffy feathers at its end dangles around the jowl. They wear sheer long black vests over the white *Gyugori*, fabric socks tied inside of their trousers, *Bagy*, and traditional straw knitted shoes. A regiment of eyes are watching us. The two maids, holding both my arms, usher me from the taxi and into the paraquin. It has small square doors on either side that are formed by strings of suspended colorful beads. Inside it there is a large red cushion embroidered with feathers and flowers. Some women approach the paraquin door, cleaving apart the dangling beans with their hands to peek in to see me. Some are mute; some exclaim "Wow!" If I just sit with my eyes cast down and in silence, they will say I am the best bride. I do.

Four men carry me over a narrow footpath. I fancy ancient Egypt, where Queen Cleopatra in the paraquin hailed her worshipping people. I do not have an audience like hers, but sunrays slanting through the open windows warm my lap and a breath of early summer air wafts pine fragrance to my nose. I see only the lower part of the trunks of the red pines here and there, and the green bushes of baby pines covering the red earth. I feel rolling hills and hear the four men panting. The further we go, the more my nervousness escalates. I seem to visit a feudal lord in his castle. I know the families are joyfully waiting for us. What do I have to be in a panic about?

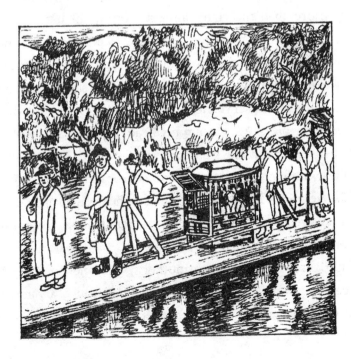

And now I am in a dark hall, where stands the ancestors' roster
chest. This black chest is opened to reveal the names of your daddy's
ancestors written with a black brush on a long scroll of white mulberry paper. The paper is folded many times, showing the long heritage I have now entered. Before the chest is a table crowded with
food and fruit, an offering to those ancestors. I sit with my eyes cast
down before the table in my wedding attire, supported by my two
bridesmaids. The hall is crowded with families and guests elbowing
one another; I can hear the women whispering about me. Your oldest
uncle—wearing our traditional garment of a long white coat—
kindles candles and burns sticks of incense. I bow and bow and bow.
I just follow my two bridal maids' guidance.

Soon after the ritual, I am led to your daddy's grandmother's
bedroom. She is eighty-five; for the past few years she can sit but is
unable to stand up and walk. She wears our conventional white blouse
and long skirt of ramie cloth that looks so comfortable and cool. She
is a very tiny figure with a round face and fair complexion; her left
eye sags more than the right, almost closed, yet her nose stands
straight. She is comely and dignified. I bow to her and sit downcast in
silence. She asks the maids to bring me next to her and holds my
hands, shaking them a few times back and forth; she peers at my face
and lifts my chin to observe me, saying, "You are Sung Hi's wife!" She
gives me many blessings, patting my head. She appears to rejoice in
our marriage. What really strikes me is her voice. I never expected
such a clear, authoritative, vigorous voice from a lady who is not only
eight-five years old but disabled. Hyun A, her voice is just like your
daddy's. I have never tired of hearing your daddy's voice—manly,
reverberating, and crystal.

After that I am ushered to another room where a feast of rain-
bow-colored savory foods and fruits are beautifully arranged on a
low table. Your grandmother already sits on the floor, cross-legged,

on one side of the table. I bow to her with the help of my two bridesmaids. She smiles with joy without a word. She sits erect; her spine is
straight. Her large features remind me of Buddha's. After she leaves,
your numerous great uncles, uncles, and aunts take her place. Every
time the seat is exchanged, I bow and bow and bow. The rituals go on
and on; it grows dark. It is time to retire....

§   §   §

The day has been arduously long. I have felt as if it will never
come to an end. But at last the growing gloom allows the day's activities to end. When my maids take me to my bedroom, throngs of
family—your daddy's many great aunts, aunts, sisters, sisters-in-law,
little nephews and nieces, and prominent female villagers—are
packed in the room and receive me with a jubilant welcome. They
introduce themselves:

"It is a long day for you!"

"I am Sung Hi's great aunt."

"I am Sung Hi's aunt, the sister of his father...."

Hyun A, I am stunned by the family's surpassing beauty and by
their well-formed features. When your daddy's sisters walk toward
me, wearing the traditional Korean long dresses of light aqua and
violet and holding closed the skirt's side edge, they look as if they are
walking down the aisle of a beauty contest—tall, lovely, slim, raven-
haired, and beautifully dressed.

Now some children are calling me, "New aunt, new aunt!" Little
ones rub my dress and some slump down on my lap, competing with
each other. The elders pull them out of my lap. There is no way for
me to tell who belongs to whom. Your daddy's older sister and the
other two sisters bring the supper table along with the teapot tray
and the fruit tray. The crowd walks out of the room, leaving the three
sisters. They pour tea in the tea cup; the oldest sister lifts my spoon

and puts it into my right hand: "Well, eat! You must be hungry," she says. "All day you didn't eat!" The youngest sister peels apples and oranges. Hyun A, I am really hungry. You would not believe the food on the table—the artfully displayed, sumptuous varieties of dishes, the delicious smells! The oysters are as big as children's palms, like abalone. The sisters urge me to take more and more. Do you remember, however, what your grandmother exhorted me to do before I came here? I eat only a little.

After they take away the dining table from my room, they allow me to have some time to rest. By tradition, your daddy is not permitted to stay or sleep with his bride; he has to stay in the men's quarters to receive male guests and stay and sleep with them for three days. So his sisters come and try to comfort me and to help me feel close to their family. Your oldest aunt tells me that tomorrow's main event for your daddy and me will be the visitation to our ancestors' tombs. To prepare me, she gives me a brief history of her ancestors:

> Our Manghori village is unique, wealthier and larger than common villages. It consists of only one tribe, the Gungju Rhee tribe, which originated from the same forefather, Rhee, Yikjae Kong, who was a prime minister at the time of the regime of the Rhee Dynasty. The villagers took great pride in him, and in his honor they built in the center of the village a shrine that contains a fine portrait. The entire village offers tribute to Yikjae Kong annually at that shrine. And they use the shrine as a gathering place for meetings and conferences.

> A hundred and fifty years ago our great-great grandfather became the governor of our province. He exercised power and wisdom for the people of our province for his lifetime.

He was buried in the Gurim, thirty miles away from this village. Our great grandparents, our grandfather, and our father lie in our mountain just behind our house; today the litter bearers carried you over that mountain.

Our great-grandfather was a well-known scholar and landlord, as well an influential leader of the village. Our grandfather was a poet, landlord, and a sage of our village. Our father was a man of character and an enlightened man who had wonderful vision. First and foremost, he was a shrewd businessman; anything he touched brought him fortune. I remember when I was in Asahi Girls' High School in Kwangju, the capital of our province, we lived in the biggest house in the city. He greatly emphasized education, not only his own children's, but for other children in the village. Our families are well educated; even under the thirty-six years of Japanese rule before the end of World War II, when that oppressive government denied education to the Korean people, our brothers and sisters received a fine education. Our family has always cared deeply about learning.

Now I want you to rest....

She gives me a goodnight smile and closes the door behind her. I am alone in the room. The night deepens by degrees. From the male quarters and the front court, the sound of footsteps and people's voices fade away, the echo of the women's footsteps in the pantry hall is silenced. Now stillness, deathly stillness, falls upon the earth.

In the morning I dress carefully in our costume—a long dress of green and red with white cloth socks; I walk through the hallway to the room where the grandmother and mother-in-law and aunts who came from other towns have spent the night. They all are already up and arrayed in their fine attire. I greet them, offering a regular bow—I bend my right leg to the floor, turn my hands back, and gracefully drop my head. "Did you have a good night?" asks the grandmother. "You must have been exhausted last night." I sit with them for a while, listening to them; then I stand up and retreat backward, facing them, and shut the door quietly. In the pantry several women with the sisters-in-law are preparing breakfast for the guests. I greet them and try to help, but they stop me, saying, "Oh, no, no, the bride must rest!"

Another fine day favors us. Your great uncles, uncles, and your daddy, with only three women—my two bridesmaids and me—go to your ancestors' tombs that lie around the foot of the mountain. We all walk to the mountain. Your oldest uncle leads us first to your great-great grandparents' tomb, then your great-grandfather's, finally your grandfather's. Each tomb's yard is well maintained—the wild grasses are mowed, the turf is evenly green, the tall marble tombstones, inscribed with the epitaphs, are polished brightly. As your aunt told me last night, your daddy's family hires a professional mountain watcher who lives with his family near the mountain; he takes care of the mountain as well as the ancestors' tombs all year round.

Each lot is located in a different sunny spot facing south. In each lot a few yellow dandelions smile at us here and there; new silver-green leaves of mugworts dot the grass sporadically; a white butterfly flutters near us. At the rim, tall pine trees cast their shadow on the lot; two orioles call to each other with tuneful voices from the pines. In the center of each lot, the husband and wife—grandmother and grandfather—lie side by side. Their resting-place is marked by the tomb, the six-foot-high tombstone that carried the epitaph, and the marble slab of the offering table that lies before the tombstone. Your daddy and I stand side by side before the offering table. I bow with the help of my two bridesmaids just as I did at the wedding ceremony. But the man's bow is a little different. He holds his hands together at his brow and kneels down on the turf and bends down until his hands touch the ground.

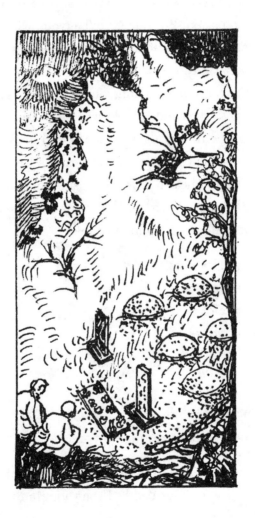

We visit your grandfather's tomb last. As I stand before this tomb, my feelings of unease and fear are transformed into rejoicing. I sit down on the grass cross-legged and bow, and a puff of wind sweeps my face as if I hear a voice whisper, "With Sung Hi, live happily forever!" I hold my hands tight, resisting the maids pulling at my elbows to lift me, and stay on the ground. I am overwhelmed by the feeling of your grandfather's presence and blessing. Everyone thinks I have fainted from weariness. When I get up, everyone shows signs of relief. Everyone is hushed. But I never tell anyone what has happened to me. Since then your grandfather's warm, fatherly spirit, securing my life with your daddy, has never left me.

In the late afternoon, your aunt Gum Myo brings a gramophone to my room, cranks the handle, and turns on a record. The sound of music floods the room. Your daddy stops by and sings with his sister. Among all the recorded songs, both like best the Japanese love song, "Memories." You have heard your daddy sing this many times; at a party, when his turn comes to sing, he always sings this love song. If I paraphrase it, it will go something like this:

> Memories, memories!
> On my blue dress suit
> I see the trace of your lipstick
> And tears of yours.
>
> I am alone, crying of
> Memories of our love.
> It is raining, and another
> Spring is here without you.

Hyun A, remember what your grandmother said before I left home? I can't flirt with your daddy. I can't join in the singing. But I remember the words always.

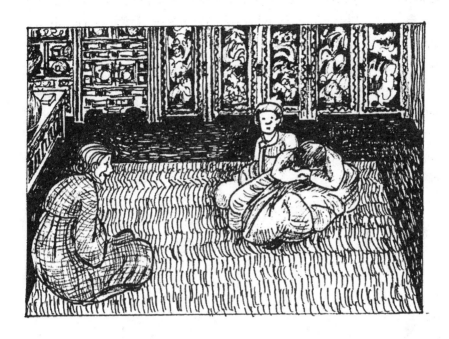

On the third day after our arrival, we walk back along the ridge of the mountain on the path where I was carried three days ago. Then our taxi rolls away, further and further from the waving hands of family and friends until the curve of the hill blocks them. The family is so kind and the home near the high mountains and the Yung Am Sea is so beautiful. But I feel fortunate that I don't have to stay there to live for my lifetime; I can come out to live in the wider world any way I choose.

—5—

Your Beginnings

Dear Hyun A,

After seven months of the joy of our new home—creamy, bright—one morning I suddenly feel sick; from then on the very smell of food makes me feel nauseous. Food is detestable even to look at, since it makes me so sick. It's unfortunate that the joy of a coming child often begins this way. The morning sickness gets worse day by day, and I can keep nothing down. Your daddy does not know what to do to help me; he goes to your grandmother at Gae Rim Dong, Kwangju, to ask for her help. She stays with us and tries to alleviate the symptoms: she eliminates the spicy or smelly foods and cooks for me light, liquid foods like rice-gruel, thin broth of soybean sprout, chicken, and beef; she grinds apples and pears and puts them into separated gauze; holding the edge of the gauze with each hand, she twists the fabric in opposite directions, squeezing the juice from them. My symptoms become aggravated notwithstanding; finally, I am so weak I can hardly teach. For that reason, I visit my obstetrician, Dr. Kim, who recommends my admission to the hospital for intravenous fluid and rest. "Your condition is serious," she says.

"I don't want to miss teaching my class because of my pregnancy," I say. "Let me try to go to school today; if I am not able, I'll return to you."

"All right, then," she says, "I'll give you quick, temporary energy: 50% glucose, 50 cc intravenously." She ties my left upper arm with a tourniquet and pokes my vein with a long needle. She advises me to take medication to alleviate my symptoms, but I hesitate to accept it because I don't know how the medicine will affect the baby. Without it, I barely make it through the following days at school. Then suddenly—within three weeks-the repulsion for food is gone as precipitously as it came.

I notice that with my pregnancy, everyone's attitude toward me is changed: whatever I do that swerves from the norm—such as over-spending—is allowed; whatever I desire to eat, even if the food is rare or difficult to get—is obtainable. I develop a kind of pica—an uncontrollable desire for sour, rare fruits such as Mogae, a fruit that has a mango-like shape but an acidic flavor. Pickled plums, pome-granates—these are on my dining table. Also I want fried whole spring chicken without batter, the gourmet dish in the Prince Chinese Res-taurant. Not only does my family give me the most beautiful fruits but the freshest ones. Our family's changing attitudes are not limited to foods. They volunteer to do my work. "Don't do it," they say, "it is too hard for you. Rest for the baby's sake."

All the family's concerns are centered on the coming baby. They try to provide me with nutritious foods and the freshest vegetables coming directly from their own gardens. I must not eat leftovers but must always have clean, fresh foods. I must not eat pork. I must have the best seat at any place. I must walk in the center of the road like a princess. Thus I am convinced that a child's education does not begin from the time of a baby's birth but from the time of the baby's conception. The experience makes me think this: when the paternal and maternal germ cells unite and begin multiple cell division, form the organs of the fetus, and grow as a fetus for the full nine months within the mother's womb, the fetus must get nutrition from his mother through the same blood via the umbilical cord. Therefore, the fetus is totally and directly dependent on the mother before his birth. Whatever the mother eats, does, and thinks, the fetus gets the same effect on his body and his mind. Even though he is unborn and unseen, he is always with his mother and is growing like a visible baby. Hyun A, that conclusion commands me to control my mind: think fairly, act restrainedly, and be pleasant and happy, as your family would say, "For the baby's sake!"

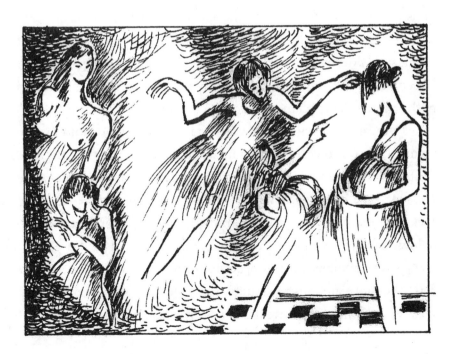

By Korean tradition, every family desires to have a baby boy more than a baby girl. This is because the boy will carry on the family name and become the master of the household. However, I am not concerned about the baby's gender but only want a perfect healthy baby.

Hyun A, when you start to kick my abdomen, I feel part of a mystic creation which is followed by an explicable joy that only a woman can experience! As my body becomes heavier month by month, your daddy hires a young woman who lives with us to do the housework and cook for us as well. The long day of standing and teaching, especially the long walk from the teacher's room up to the second floor to the classroom, causes my ankles to swell and causes me to move slowly. For support I girdle my abdomen tightly with several yards of white cloth.

Hyun A, in the later part of my pregnancy my mother occasionally boils and simmers the roots of *Duduk* (*Codonopsis Lanceolata*) and *Doragee* (a broad bellflower), plants that grow in the mountains. Before she cooks them, she blends them with fowl or carp. They taste terrible—blah, bitter, queasy, and medicinal. But I eat them, surrendering to your grandmother's love and sincerity for us. "Rhee Sil A [she calls me customarily the Rhee's lady] this makes both a mother and a child strooooong." She stresses the word "strong."

I prepare your clothes, blankets, and a wide, long cloth binder made of cotton to carry you on my back. At the same time my students, who are senior high school girls, make all sorts of things for you with their own hands: infant's clothes either for boys or for girls, socks, quilts, bonnets, caps.... Among the gifts, your black velvet pillow that is embroidered with colorful silk thread in flower patterns with little birds is too beautiful to use. The closer to my due date, the more anxious my students are for the baby to come. Your great grandfather—my grandfather—gives you the name "Hyun A," which means wise and elegant beauty (should you be a girl!). The joys of preparation and expectation make ready for the coming of the baby as the seed of a plant is made ready to sprout under the spring breath and spring showers.

Hyun A, during the whole course of pregnancy, one thing that is hard to ignore is my fear, fear caused by uncertainty of the baby's development, fear that the baby will not be perfect. The fear attaches to me as my shadow follows me under light. This fear sits in my deepest recesses; it is uttered only in my prayers. The closer the due day is, the stronger it becomes.

I decide to stay with your Yung Am grandmother—your daddy's mother who came to us two weeks ahead of my due day—for home delivery, not delivery at the hospital. I will not have a doctor. Your grandmother had seven children of her own; besides she has many other grandchildren and is as knowledgeable as is a midwife. I myself have knowledge about childbirth. The women in my family had no specific problems with childbirth. If any complication should take place, your daddy is right by us to take care of us; and the hospital is located not far from us. The house is far cleaner than the hospital, having less exposure to germs.

I work at the school right up until labor starts. When the pains come at three- to five-minute intervals, I feel I am hearing a fanfare of trumpets for the long-awaited battle. The excitement, along with fear of battle itself, sweeps my mind. My mother-in-law takes a bath and changes into clean clothes and squats toward her Buddhist Temple in the south side of the Yung Am district. She recites her prayers by heart, rubbing her palms together in a circular motion. When my pains get harder, she thinks the delivery will be soon and asks your daddy to leave the room. This is our timeless custom. I don't know what your daddy will do while I am passing through the long travail. However I watched a western movie titled *Montogane* when I was a teenager. Someplace in Africa, the hero goes to a nearby river when his wife is in labor; he swims countless laps without pausing until his wife has had his baby.

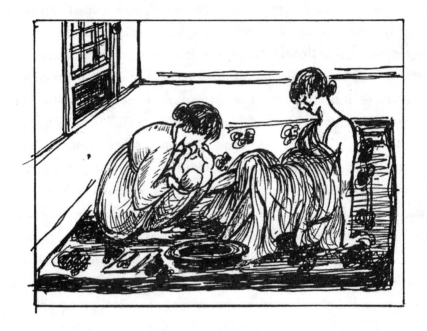

Your grandmother is wrong. The delivery is *not* soon. The accelerated labor lasts hour after hour, ever increasing in intensity, and the contractions come regularly every two or three minutes. I try not to use any pain medication. I kneel on the floor and put my face into my quilt to muffle my noisy moans. Every time the pain comes, my knees rub around over the floor; both hands grip a part of the quilt; my groans stifle away into the quilt. Your grandmother sits by me; as the pain comes, she holds either my shoulders or arms: "Daughter, daughter, just be patient," she says. "It won't be long." As the pain leaves, she wipes my sweat-drenched face and smoothes back my disheveled hair. She sometimes pretends to fan my face with her open bare hand. "Amya [the name for the child's mother], Amya, muster your courage! Push, push push, push harder! Blow, breathe, blow, blow, breathe! That's it!"

Finally she senses that the baby really is coming down soon. She checks her instruments on the steel tray—a pair of boiled scissors, two five-inch braids of thick sewing thread, and several pieces of sterilized gauze. After a few incredibly propelling pains, amniotic fluid gushes out through the burst membranes; I lie back and with one last rending pain, you glide out into your grandmother's hands. You are crying hard, almost screaming. Your grandmother is tying your umbilical cord; the girl is sent for your daddy. "Good heavens!" your grandmother cries, "my Amya, the baby is a girl, a healthy, pretty girl!" When your daddy dashes into the room, your grandmother hands you to him. "O, oh, ohh..." holding you in his arms and rocking you up and down, he merely makes noisy exclamations; he cannot put words into a sentence. About seven minutes later, another squeezing cramp comes. "Amya, once more give a push!" says your grandmother. The bulky, glistening purplish-blue afterbirth slides down on the floor accompanied by a pool of blood. My mound of abdomen collapses into a small, hard basketball below the umbilicus. Your grandmother changes my sweat-soaked blouse and blood-smeared skirt for clean ones, and she mops and cleans the room. "Amya, you worked hard!" she says. "You endured the travail better than anybody else I know of!" She caresses my hair a few times with genuine warm affection. "Aygo! [oh my goodness] You are hungry!"

"I'd rather sleep!" I reply.

Then your daddy hands you into my arms. There is nothing to match that moment of joy in all this world. I forget those tormenting pains all the night through. I check all your fingers and unfold the swath to examine your whole body. "Thank God! You are a perfectly healthy baby!" I mutter to myself. I heave a sigh of relief. I feel I am holding an unreachable star in my arms! You are tiny, about six and a half pounds, but so strong and splendid! Your eyes are swollen even worse than mine; they are closed but occasionally open, showing black, gleaming pupils. You cry with widely opened mouth, wielding two tiny fists in the air; your strong little feet are kicking the baby blanket. The white greasy vernix covers your entire body, even your long black hair. It is not surprising that you could float for a full nine months in the water of the amniotic sac!

After settling down from the exciting moment of your birth, I sense that my knees are sore. I look at them; they ooze with blood. After going through this travail, I would seem to be able to endure any kind of severe pain.

I can hear the male servant anxiously ask the girl who is helping your grandmother for charcoal. By Korean tradition, when a household has a new child, we put outside the porch door a straw rope that is pierced by red dried pepper and fragments of charcoal. From the rope hangs a long white piece of mulberry paper, 2" by 5"; a piece of pine twig; and pieces of bamboo leaves—all these are arrayed alternately down the length of the straw rope. This shows people that the house has a newborn baby. If the baby is a girl, red peppers will not be put on the straw rope. This emblem gives a warning to people, saying, "If anyone has any disease, is sick, or is not clean, please don't enter this house!"

Your grandmother takes you from my arms; she bathes you in warm water in a round, portable bathtub. Your daddy tries to help her work by holding you. When I hold you again in my arms, the blazing morning sun is rising up; it brightens our room and blesses you. The clustered red persimmons bend their branches with sparse, dry leaves at the back and the front yard. I can hear the daily activities of the morning: the train is rushing on the rails and whistling clamorously in the air; the neighbor's dogs bark resonantly; the morning cocks crow proudly as if announcing your birth to the world.

You are born at 8:40 a.m. on November 6, 1957.

God, hear my prayer!

Praise Thy name:
As I hold our own child in my hands,
I do not stop to think—of their own accord
My lips, my eyes are towards Thee,
Gazing to Thee on high, uttering to Thee:
Thank you, God, for bestowing to us
This healthy, perfect child of ours!

Praise Thy creation:
Through this childbirth
Thy words, Thy presence, Thy love and grace
Reveal themselves as true to me
As my own breath.

What Thou told men—Thou created a man in Thy image—
Is beyond doubt because our child has our own image.
Thou rejoiced greatly in Thy creation
As Thou overlooked Thy creation of the universe
And a man. I now understand Thy joy
As I hold my child, this little creation of my own.

Praise Thy grace:
Thou let me be a woman
To realize its exclusive privilege
Being the mother of a child!
My grumbles to Thee would say this:
Why have you made me a girl
So that I have to do chores of the house
All the time, all the time?
Now they are evaporated and gone!

Praise Thy blessings:
Before Thee
I hold this our child;
I consecrate her to Thee.
Bless her with Thy hands of love!

Thy blessings make her bind to Thee,
Her lips to praising Thy name,
Her eyes to gazing up to Thy light,
Her ears to listening to Thy truth.
Thy blessings are her life forever.

§   §   §

After a baby is born, the involution—the restoration of the uterus—has to take place. The uterine muscle fibers stretch five hundred times their normal size during the nine months of pregnancy; after the baby's delivery, they gradually return to their original state. The process takes six weeks, unlike stretched rubber that returns at once when released from tension. By timeless Korean tradition, an ideal atmosphere for the mother during involution is a warm temperature without any draft. For that reason, even in summer—and of course in winter—the room temperature should be kept warm, and the mother ought to wear warm clothes and even put on cloth socks. Her food must be hot too, such as our hot seaweed soup with sea foods like high-protein hard-shelled mussels. Seaweed contains a lot of iodine as well as coagulants that can reduce bleeding and facilitate involution. When I take this hot soup with hot rice, my face is bathed in dripping, rainy sweat; however, I am not allowed to open the door nor change into lighter clothes. I notice a heat rash on my back and brow, but I have neither joint pains nor back pains nor other problems. My milk flows bountifully for the baby; most of the time it wets my clothes. The breast-feeding, too, facilitates involution.

After the baby is born, our household alters greatly. All the family's attention focuses on the baby; this new member in the family makes the house busy and noisy with the baby's crying, with more cooking, cleaning, and washing than before. This responsibility for our newly created life means harder work and tender care. It seems to be true that good things are not acquired without suffering and struggle.

The family's indulgence toward me continues just as during my pregnancy. I don't have to work at any house chores; I can just take it easy and eat good food and feed my baby. Both of your grandmothers stay with me in turn, doing all the chores with the maid. They do not allow me spicy foods. Throughout the puerperal period the following recipes are repeated intermittently for the baby's nursing and for the restoration of my health: Ginseng roots with big carps are boiled and simmered; Condonopsis Lanceolata's roots with chicken plus dried dates and chestnuts are boiled and simmered; sometimes roots of broad bellflowers with beef are boiled and simmered. The food I eat is like medicine for you and for me.

By Korean tradition the third-day celebration is special, because if the mother and baby survive up to the third day, they are most likely to be all right to continue their lives. For this reason, your grandmother bathes in the early morning, changes to clean white clothes, and prepares for the tribute to the spirits of our ancestors and the Buddha. She gives them thanks for the safety of both mother and baby through pregnancy and delivery. In addition she asks them to give their blessings to the mother and baby and to all the family.

Your grandmother puts a handful of clean straw on the floor of the western wall of the room, since the Buddha's temple in the Wyul Choos Mountain at Yung Am Town faces toward the west. A white bowl filled with clear spring water is placed in the middle of the spread straw. In a large ceramic steamer (two feet by three feet) is a

sweet rice cake in many layers interspersed with red beans; she lifts
the steamer by the handles and places it in front of the spread straw.
The cake has steamed all night; its delicious aroma fills the room.
Finally she squats just at the back of the straw and begins muttering
and rubbing her hands around, palm to palm. "Spirits of our ancestors and Buddha, thank your for your protection of both mother and
baby. Bless them bountifully with health, wealth, and many more
children." She continues whispering in different words but with the
same rubbing of her palms for another ten minutes. After that she
cuts the cake and shares the happy occasion with neighbors, friends,
relatives and the family.

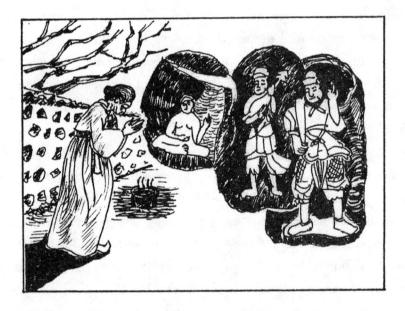

On the third night after your birth, as it grows dim and stars
appear in the sky, your grandmother piles dry wood at the corner of
the front yard, builds a fire, and burns the afterbirth to ash. Once the
creation of life is completed through the afterbirth, that organ is no
longer needed; it must go with the fire.

When I first begin breast-feeding, I am uncomfortable before your daddy and your grandmothers. I open a door and go into a small room attached to the main room; there I stay and feed the baby. However, your grandmother notices me and says, "Do not be ashamed of feeding the hungry baby before the family; you ought to feel pride and joy in feeding her." Despite her wise advice, it takes me a while to do this because to expose myself to such an extent is hard for me. As I hold you in my arms to quench your hunger, I look down at your face suckling the nipple; you close your eyes and open your right hand and try to grab the breast. You take gulp after gulp, making chirping sounds like music. Looking at you, I feel satisfied that you have abundant milk. Sometimes too much milk and too quick gulping make you choke and stop suckling. Sometimes unexpectedly, in the middle of the feeding, you stop suckling and sleep soundly and breathe hard, then again suckle a few times and sleep with the nipple in your mouth. I see peaceful features—nothing to be worried about—your nose is round, fair, well-formed like your daddy's; your small scarlet lips and crimson cheeks are like a seraph's. I imagine this moment is the true living picture in the large frame. I feel this moment is an inseparable bond between you and me, physically, mentally and spiritually. This is the mystery of life's creation and continuum. This is the woman's privilege. A mother and a child are bound inseparably; no one can break this tie.

After delivery, four weeks pass swiftly. Hyun A, you grow fast and well every day, as in the spring the new buds rapidly grow from the first pink swell to the burst of green. The umbilical cord dries and drops off, leaving a depressed, clean scar. You now lift your head on your own, and you focus on me eye to eye, trying to smile. My body grows stronger and recovers. It is hard to rest two more weeks at home because I am the senior class teacher who is in charge of the class and must prepare for the many special events of their graduation. This is the critical period for my class.

Today is the first day to go back to work. I awake early in the morning and look outside. It is snowing; the snow is thinly piled upon the black branches of the persimmon trees and the green arms of the cedars like white flowers and on the roofs and ground like white sheets. From the leaden sky the snow flakes—wafery, small, large—fly dizzily and alight aslant on the earth without sound. No one hears the sifting of the particles which fill the cold space and fall endlessly down, searching for their own places. As the wind lays down its wings, everything is still but for the clouds of smoke rising from the thatch houses. Looking to the east, I see the bright sun ascend; its light stops the snow; it warms the earth and prepares me for my first day of work.

—6—

Struggle for Two Roles

Dear Hyun A,

Combining breast feeding a baby and teaching students in a high school is really difficult. However, the baby's first year is the important foundation for that baby's life. During that period, the most desirable food for her health is mother's milk. For mother's milk contains a variety of immune bodies as well as highly balanced nutrients.

Before I return to work—four weeks after the delivery—your daddy serendipitously discovers that his great-uncle Yung Sam, your grandfather's second cousin, lives just across the street from the school. His home is behind Dr. Kang's office of dermatology. The great-uncle is a truck driver; the great-aunt is a housewife. They are in their late sixties and have three grown children who have all gone from home. They generously accept your daddy's proposal that they provide a place to feed our baby from Monday to Friday and a half day on Saturday. Maid Hyun Bok, my cousin, brings you from our home one hour later than I leave home, and she stays at the great-uncle's during the daytime and watches you; in the after-noon, she carries you back home one hour earlier than I leave the school. Our house is over two miles away from the school; I have to walk more than half an hour to the school. At that time the only transportation vehicles were our feet.

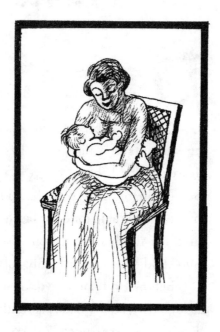

I teach one hour for every class, with ten minutes between classes and a forty-five-minute lunch break. I am able to adjust this teaching schedule to my breast-feeding. Your first year, during the day, is spent at your great-uncle Yung Sam's being fed, being changed, turning over, crawling around, teething, reeling to stand, staggering to step, and jabbering: *Agim* (aunt), *Halabugy* (grandfather), *Halmuny* (grandmother), *Appa* (daddy), and *Umma* (mother). Sometimes, my students beg me to see the baby during lunchtime. They come like a school of fish with toys, dolls, clothes, socks, mittens and other little things for the baby. They make everything by hand. They love the baby; sometimes without reason they scream, "Yah, the baby, let's go see her!"

"She is the cutest baby we have ever seen!"

"Teacher Yoo, can we take her home?"

When I am tied up with a teachers' meeting or at the physics laboratory, my breasts swell and becomes hard as a rock, giving me rending pain; this pain assails me with an inexplicable deep down sadness, as though it were the call of my hungry baby's crying.

One day your Aunt Ho Jung Mumma tells me that she met Hyun Bok, who carried you piggyback through the heavy snow; your face was covered with a long cape. She felt so worried that she opened the cape to see the three-months-old baby, but your wide-awake, beautiful, and vibrant features wiped away any feeling of concern for you.

When you are around seven months old, my baby sister Yun Sung visits us, saying, "Wow, the baby is so beautiful! She is so healthy and happy; no crying and not a fretful baby at all! Elder sister Chi Sun, what's your secret?'

"There is no secret, my baby sister!" She does not know how hard the baby's mother has struggled silently day and night for the baby's health and happiness.

When you are eight to nine months old, the muggy, sweltering summer evenings come—no houses are equipped with air conditioners, and in the dark the pernicious mosquitoes are rampant around the houses. Beside the *Pyung Sang,* (the wide bamboo low-legged chair on which all the family can sit), the men build a smoking fire of green grass to chase those mosquitoes away. But your daddy figures out another, better way to lull you: he holds you and walks to the railroad tracks a quarter mile away from our house. No matter how sultry the night is, at the railroad there are no poisonous insects; there ever blows the cool summer breeze. He rocks you and lulls you by the soft breath and brings you home, saving you from the insects' biting.

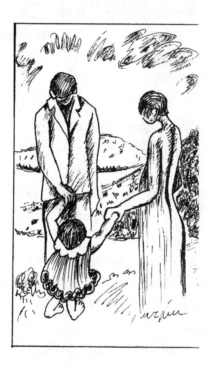

One of the greatest merits of the Korean family system is that we help one another when help is needed. But for the help of our great uncle and great aunt, I might have chosen cow's milk rather than mother's milk for our child. Both your grandmothers love your daddy and me, and they extend their unconditional love to you, too, as if they live only for us.

—7—

Medical School?

Dear Hyun A,

Now you are three years old, and your daddy and I have a wonderful family life: we have built a new home near your daddy's Chosun University; your daddy has just been promoted to associate professor in his Physics Department; I have a teaching job at the Kwangju Girls High School; Korea is settling down from the ravages of the Korean War politically and economically. Your daddy and I are thinking of having another baby.

It is a summer evening after dinner. I open the window of our study; the sweet mountain breeze puffs in and out of the room. I go to my desk and draw a few diagrams of female organs on large drawing paper; some of them are marked with colors to distinguish them from others. Tomorrow I am going to substitute in class for the American Army nurse, who usually gives a special lecture to all the senior classes once a week at the high school. The subject will be about female physiology, especially the menstrual cycle.

Your daddy comes into the room. "Wow! That is an excellent sketch. I didn't know you are good at drawing. Do you still think of becoming a doctor?" he asks.

"Yes, I do! This is not for my class but for the lecture usually given by the American Army nurse, Nancy Morgan. The principal wants me to substitute for her."

"You can go to medical school. I'll support you if you want to," he says.

"Really?" I reply no further than that.

He turns out of the room. But he threw a stone in the calm lake of my mind. I can see a yielding ripple; it's growing bigger and bigger, disturbing the entire tranquil lake. I feel as if my tranquil life is over. I have always wanted to go to medical school since I was a nursing student in high school. However, I have a job, I am married, I have a baby. I have been carried away with the comfort of a happy family life. We are content: we decorate our new house with bright cherry-blossom wall paper and new lacy curtains and furniture—a bedroom bureau, a dining room table wrought in clam shells. In the summer I love to plant all manner of flowers—rose bushes and wild flowers all around the house. All summer long the various colors and shapes and fragrances change as one sort of flower fades away and another flower takes over.... Do you remember the wire chicken coop in our backyard? Your daddy asked one of his cousins to build it, so now you can watch and play with the chickens. White roosters with large red crests proudly crow; with their long white tail feathers, they like to swagger about the pen and dominate the hens and chicks. The white hens lay eggs every day. Your daddy and I have peace and fulfillment.

But somehow the flame of my dream to be a medical doctor has flickered all the time. Suddenly, your daddy's words, like wind on smoldering tinder, fire my whole heart. Now I am in turmoil. The excitement of fancy and impossibility to act gyrate through my mind. That night my sleepless mind becomes a spinning machine. The same thoughts eddy through my mind and confuse it; it is hard to straighten out the ideas. I get up and take out a paper and a pencil and actually jot down the things that might happen if I accept his offer:

1. Would Chonnan University Medical School accept a married woman with a child? I have never heard of such a thing.

2. Can we afford the four years financially? We can; we can manage it.

3. What about another baby? No way!

4. Can I compete with young, single medical students? It's questionable, yet there is the possibility.

5. What if both families oppose our idea; could we stand up a against their objections? We can, because they are not giving us any financial support.

6. Can I resign my teaching position? I can, because I will have a better position in the future.

This way, I obtain a clear answer: four *yeses* out of six, one *no*, one *questionable*. Therefore, if the medical school accepts me, I will become a medical student and study to become a doctor. Before the sun comes up, I decide to accept your daddy's proposal. But I say to myself, "Not now. Think again before you leap." My life surely will become different from the peaceful, happy world of the past.

Why should I go through the stormy pathway to study again at this late age? Completing medical school is the hardest task for even young college students. I am now twenty-nine. I have achieved as high a position socially and personally as I now can. The more I think in this direction, the more I tend to waver in my resolution. On the other hand, I am still not too old to start, and I have just one child, not two or three. Best of all, your daddy has volunteered to help me and let me grow. As a Korean, I cannot believe that I have such a great person as my husband. The average man would not even dream of such an idea! If I let this chance pass by, to be a medical doctor will only be a dream—an unaccomplished dream that will haunt my soul both through life and after death. This is the time, the right time, and the last chance for me! I again affirm my resolution to go to medical school. I send in my application.

I acquired the seed of the dream to be a doctor while I attended the Nursing High School affiliated with the Chonman University Medical School. We nursing students were required to have poly-clinic training at the Medical School Hospital. We learned clinical nursing at every department in the hospital. A young female patient was brought by stretcher from the emergency room to the Obstet-rics and Gynecology Department; she was dying. No one, not even the registered nurses, were capable of saving her. But the doctors took her to surgery and operated at once, and they saved her life. A trauma patient with badly broken bones in his legs was brought to the Orthopedic Department; the doctors operated on him and put him in a cast for six weeks; we saw him walk out with a limp. Patients came struggling to breathe with heart or lung disease; the doctors gave them medicine that relieved their symptoms. Doctors appeared to me to be magicians or angels or gods, curing the sick and easing their suffering. I thought, "What an important, sacred job they have!" I thought I could help patients more as a doctor than as a nurse.

Someday, I wanted to put on a white gown and put a stethoscope in my pocket and see patients, diagnosing their exact problems and prescribing medicine or performing a Cesarean section that would save a baby and mother. I loved to watch *authorities*, professors, the chiefs of each department. I envied the authorities their omniscient knowledge and skills

And now almost two months have passed since I applied for medical school. In the late summer, the cicadas hide in the tall persimmon trees and shrill out in the hot afternoon; the grains of rice in the fields are filling their golden husks, bending their heads down; the green-brown locusts fly about in the rice patches.

One afternoon in this season, I receive a letter from the dean of the medical school: "At our last faculty meeting, we all agreed to allow you to take the entrance examination to be a medical student."

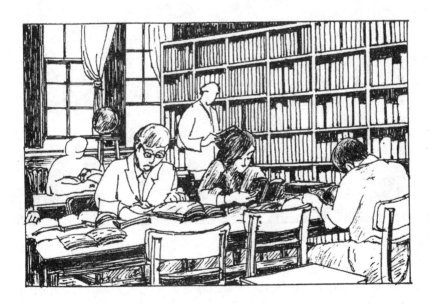

Two weeks later I receive another letter from the dean of the medical school: "Congratulations! You passed the entrance examination for becoming a student in the Class of 1959 at Chonnam University Medical School. The class will begin on March 1, 1959." After receiving the letter, there is no choice left but to enter medical school.

I have six months to prepare before beginning classes. In my mind I hear a bugle that blows for battle.

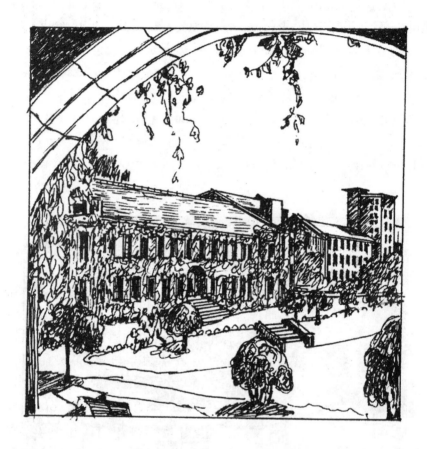

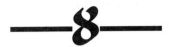

Medical School!

Dear Hyun A,

Following the graduation of my senior class of the Kwangju Girls High School around the end of February 1959, I hand in my resignation to white-haired Principal Shin, who is alone in his office. I respect his cleverness, his administrative ability. He speaks to me with concern:

"Are you sure? Even now, if you change your mind, you can take the letter back. You know how hard it is to fill your position nowadays! Teacher Yoo, do you realize how difficult it will be to complete medical school as a married woman with a child? Most likely you will succeed, but you might possibly fail. I'll hold this letter for one more day. Think about this once more!" he gives me his sincere, fatherly advice.

"Thank you, Principal Shin, for your concern as well as for everything you have done for me.

But I do not regret my decision," I answer him in a trembling voice.

"We will miss you greatly. You are a good teacher; the students speak highly of you. You have done a good job for the school. Good luck to you!" He expresses his regret at losing me. As I close his door, I sense that I have just handed in my precious treasurers—my students, my position in the school—to a stranger. Most of my colleagues think that I have lost my senses: "Imagine, twenty-nine years of age and a lady with dependents!" They feel sorry for me.

But Ok Za Kim, the piano teacher, a middle-aged spinster, rushes up to me: "Teacher Yoo, congratulations on your entrance to medical school! How I envy your courage! I wanted to go to graduate school for a doctorate in music; then I could be a professor in a university. Yet I never cut the Gordian knot, and I will be a high school teacher until I retire. Well, I don't have a strong will and courage like you. Here, the teachers are saying, 'She is crazy to give up her good job.' But in their hearts they envy you. You are not crazy; you move in the right direction. You will make your dream come true; I have faith in you. However, we will all miss you."

She adds some strength to my determination to move up against the general stream of opposition as the salmon stream up to their destiny.

Hyun A, your great-uncle, your daddy's uncle, calls on us and asks your daddy, "Sung Hi Ya, is it true that you intend to send your wife to medical school?" His pale, stern face is swollen with rage and is as gray as his long Korean coat.

"Yes, Uncle, that is true."

"How in the world did you come up with such a crazy idea, sending your wife to medical school and allowing her to give up her respected, secure job? Even a young, single man faces a hard time in completing medical school. Do you think she can take four years of schooling? You must be out of your mind!" he shrills out in fury. "Your brothers can't understand your foolishness!" In his fury he holds his hat in his left hand and flicks the brim with his forefinger. Then he flings the door open and slams out the gate.

Hyun A, my brother, your Uncle Gae Rim Don, also thinks your daddy is out of his mind. The two grandmothers are not angry, but they worry that I may fail. They just pray and hope that we will succeed at whatever we decide to do. I feel so bad because we have caused both your grandmas pain in their old age instead of giving them comfort. Your daddy and I are heavily pressed by other people's ridicule as well as the family's objection and anxiety. But I peer into the crystal ball and see only one solution for all this turmoil: Without fail, I must blaze a trail in becoming medical doctor.

Finally in early spring, the time has come to start school. Today's morning sky is gray, but the air is soft. Spring is awakening everywhere from its deathly winter slumber. Life germinates from the gray earth: the green baby leaves burst forth from the maple branches, the redbud trees blossom out in pink; daffodils and tulips spring from the gray ground around the houses; the fields of barley and wheat grow green; yellow dandelions are strewn brightly on the green turf. People crowd the street.

The Chonnam University Medical School Hospital is at the east of Kwangju City adjacent to the medical school campus. Our lecture building is on the campus of the hospital. It has two divided lecture rooms, one twice as large as the other. Our lecture room is the bigger one because we have 144 students in our class. The floor of the classroom is made of cement. The professor lectures from a cement platform on which is placed a magenta wooden podium. Behind him is a large blackboard. About ten feet from the podium, the room rises in tiers of cement steps like those of an outdoor stadium. Our desks are narrow planks about ten feet long set in rows that scramble up to the top of the room. Our chairs are also long, narrow wooden planks placed upon the cement steps. The north and south walls of the building are made of windows.

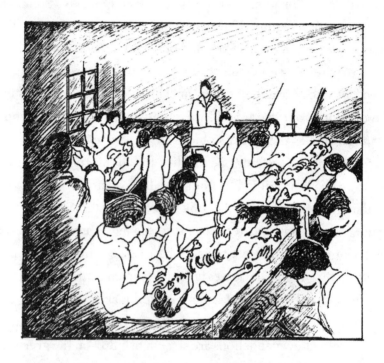

The lecture room sounds rough and cold, but the window walls make the room bright. The south-side windows are shaded by the ancient, sacred Dang San Tree; the trunk is so wide that it takes three men with open arms to circle it. The giant tree towers up and branches out broadly to the sky. The new green buds burst forth as if small heads of green flowers cover the gray branches. On the west side of the tree is a blue-gray stone monument for Shin Ik Chun, the great statesman and scholar who reigned in this province from 1605 to 1660. On it is inscribed "Chun Yearn Wan Gol" (A Millennium Stubborn Bone). It stands out as a symbol of the undying spirit of the medical school. On the south side of the tree there is a white two-storied building for the tuberculosis patients.

When I enter the classroom, many students are chattering and filling the room with noise. I can feel curious eyes on me, and the voices momentarily are hushed. Two female students among all the male students are sitting side by side at the first row of desks; they smile and wave to me. I approach them; they make room for me beside them. "Teacher Yoo, we heard you are going to study medicine. Do your remember, you taught us physics and chemistry while we were in Kangju Girls High School." "I am Gee Sun Chong"; "I am Kim Ae Sook." They smile as they speak. I smile back at them and say how glad I am to see them. But I feel odd, out of place, as though I am the one white bean among all the red beans. I feel awkward at being with the young and with my students, and perhaps somewhat degraded, but I am glad to see familiar faces.

The most difficult moment—the first meeting with my class-mates—has passed, and Professor Gun Choong Gi rushes into the room for his human anatomy class. He puts on his white gown with a few brown spots around his big pockets. He does not smile. He does not want to lose any time with jokes or welcoming words, and he plunges directly into the main subject, the human anatomy, saying, "Besides my book [in Korean], I recommend *Gray's Anatomy* to you as a reference. Anatomy is the fundamental and essential knowledge to acquire in order to be a medical doctor...."

He starts from osteology—the bony system or skeleton. His lecture continues without interruption until the last minute. Then in succession we have classes in pharmacology, physiology, and biochemistry. I buy the necessary books and go home. These are very heavy volumes to handle. The tension of facing an entirely different world on that first day makes me more exhausted than does the work involved in the classes.

§   §   §

Time passes swiftly, and now I have come almost to the end of my first year of medical school. Through the year, we have studied human anatomy: embryology, histology, osteology, the muscular and nervous systems, the blood vascular system, and the visceral system. At the final stage, we have to identify the organs and structures that we have studied from a dead human body. This process is of importance to all medical students.

The medical school morgue is in the building of the anatomy department, which is of part of the medical school complex. The complex is built around a great grass-covered square. Around the square stand many individual red-brick buildings; the administration building, the building for lectures, the building of anatomy, of pathology, of microbiology, of biochemistry, of pharmacology, and of physiology.

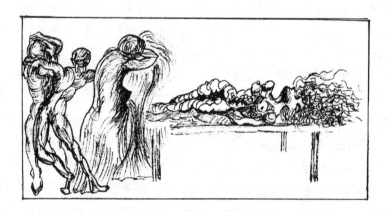

In the anatomy department there is an autopsy room for the medical students. Our class is ready: we put on our white gowns and enter the room; we see that the room has a cement floor and window walls. There are fifteen wooden tables placed side by side, and on each table is a corpse covered with a white sheet. The formalin-soaked, wrinkled, pale soles of the corpses' feet stick out from under the sheets, and the sheets outline the figure of each corpse and droop down, covering the table legs. In the room there is nothing more. The atmosphere is silent, bleak, and eerie; and the room is filled with the fumes of the formaldehyde, which makes the stomach queasy and irritates the eyes.

The class is momentarily hushed, but Professor Gwyun is undisturbed. He divides us into fifteen groups, and his nonchalant tone and attitude make the students break their silence and start to work. We open the sheet over the corpse on each table. My group's corpse is a female who died of a brain tumor. I feel at first that I cannot do this work, but I am calmed as I look around and see the other students working. One man goes out of the room because of his vomiting and headache, but he comes back and stays until the end of the class. I think many of us feel sick at the smell and sight of the corpses.

We put on rubber gloves, and with the scalpel we cut open the scalp, face, neck, chest, and belly; eventually we tear the corpse in pieces like rags; we look like hideous scavengers. The body's debris is scattered all over the table. Eyeballs are in our hands; every organ and tissue is examined. The skull is opened by a saw used in the orthopedic department and we study the brain, preserving it in the formalin jar. In my first year of medical school I found the anatomy class the most difficult and most interesting. We have studied the brain in a model; we have studied tissue under the microscope. Now in this class we study and experience what we have learned with real substances. No one fails to finish our autopsy class. We all pay homage to the departed souls who in dying left us the precious gift of their bodies for our study that will allow us to benefit the living.

§   §   §

In my first year of medical school I give all of my time and energy to the study, learning and being tested on what I have learned. Afterwards, the school has a short summer break. Before the beginning of my second year of medical school, I am asked to come in to see Professor Hong Syung Min, Dean of the Medical School. I am not told why he wants to see me. I am apprehensive as to what I may have done wrong, and I wait nervously outside the Dean's door before I enter the office.

Professor Hong Syung Min is a nationally known ophthalmologist and one of the pioneers of corneal implantation. When I enter the room, he is alone and is engrossed in writing as if he were in the midst of something that should be done at once. He is wearing the doctor's white gown and sits in front of a large rectangular mahogany desk covered with a thick sheet of glass. On the desk there is a crystal block holding a black pen and an ink pot. Right by the crystal, a round white case containing red material for stamping his seal to sign documents is ready to use. A few thick books on ophthalmology in English are on the right corner of the desk. The fluorescent light reflects his shadow on the glass. Behind his chair stand two bright flags fringed with long golden tassels—the national Korean flag and the flag of Chonnam National Medical School.

In the center of the solid white Korean flag is the national emblem of Tae Guck, the Great Absolute, the source of Yin and Yang. This is a round circle symbolizing the round universe divided into two circular swirls: the upper red one is Yang; the lower blue one, Yin. The royal blue medical school flag has its own golden emblem with a laurel branch. On the white walls are framed pictures of the school campus and the faculty of the school. A mahogany bookshelf loaded with books occupies the left corner of the room; right next to it is a bronze bust of Hippocrates. Comfortable beige couches are placed by Professor Hong's desk. A white tea table holds a white ceramic flower vase filled with pink roses. A summer breeze wafts in and out through the window screens as though the day is breathing like men.

I keep silent for a brief moment until Professor Hong has finished writing. As I look at him, I remember something from half a dozen years ago: he was then our Nursing High School principal. I waited longingly for his Nursing Ethics class, which was held for one hour on every Monday when I was a senior in high school. I remember him not only because he taught an important subject so well but even more because of his gentle and refined and warm manner that seemed natural, like second nature. All of my other professors had manners that seemed stern, rigid, and authoritative—our customary attitude to follow. Dr. Hong's gentle manner distinguished him from the others. He smiled at us. He never raised his deep bass voice. He scolded wayward students with his smiles and gentle words, and they bent before him more quickly than they would have with harsh punishment. His strength and enchantment lay in the free flow of flexibility and the resilience of kindness. I saw him as a soft breeze among the blast of wind.

"How are you? I'm sorry I made you wait," says Dr. Hong. His gentle smile spreads over his face like a just-blown flower bud. He looks a little older, but his deep voice and fair complexion are unchanged.

"How is your study? I imagine it is truly hard for you," says he.

"Yes," I reply, "I have worked hard." After keeping silent for a moment, I tell him my real feeling:

For all the difficult conditions I face as a married woman student with a child, I find, strangely enough, that there are certain unexpected advantages. I feel secure and stable financially since I don't have to worry about paying my school tuition. I am not worried about loneliness.

Therefore, I can concentrate far more effectively on my studies. Besides, married life does not allow me much time, and so I am urged to use my limited time effectively. At the same time, I am so appreciative of my present position it allows me to aim at my dream.

After listening to me, he says, "I never thought of it that way. You are a special case.

"I called you to give you my personal congratulations on your achievement. The school scholarship committee selected several students who have reached such high records that they are qualified to receive the Korean-German Scholarship. You are one of them. Continue to strive for your dream."

He beams upon me warm fatherly affection. I am speechless, overwhelmed with joy. "Thank you," I barely say. "I'll...." I never can finish that sentence. I can hardly suppress my rapture as I leave the room.

§   §   §

Once men ride on the giant wheel of time, it rolls on by itself, and so my wheel of medical school goes on at its own pace without halting. The wheel of time brings you now to the age of five. I am in the third year of medical school. I have many subjects to study, including polyclinics. Particularly at the time of examinations, time is a crucial factor for me. Final examinations have started in this late winter.

In the middle of the week, without any warning symptoms—earache, sore throat, diarrhea, rashes, or cough—you are sick with a high fever; the thermometer shows 103 F. Why in the world in the middle of my frantic examination time should you be seriously sick? Why at this time! You have been an extraordinarily healthy baby and child, rarely sick. Why at this time! I am angry beyond frustration at what is happening, yet not at you. It is life; any kind of unpredictable accident may take place. Both you and I are helpless before those. Then, what should I do? It is plain and simple. To me, you are first and foremost, more important than any other thing, even flunking my examinations. I may take those exams again some other time, or in the worst case, I will repeat the third year once again. If anything happens to you, though—the thought is impossible! This last realization settles me down to a certain extent.

So I put all my books down. I examine you; you do not have specific sighs of tonsillitis, ear infection, or meningitis, which eases my mind. I try giving you baby aspirin first, and then an alcoholic sponge bath. I piggyback you and walk around the room with a gentle rocking motion. Your fever makes my back hot like a wrapped heated stone, and you lean on my back without making a sound. Still my mind is on my books, fretting about exams. I say to myself in a low tone, "Oh, oh, I may flunk tomorrow's exams."

"Mom, you study! I'll go back to my room and lie down by myself." You try to wriggle down from my back.

"That's all right," I say. "Mom can hold you for a while. Just put your head on Mom's back." I say this and gently rock around the room. And I think to myself, "What a thoughtful kid! Exceptional for her age!" After a time I feel on my back that your fever cools down and you sleep soundly, and so does my frustration and my fear. The next day I take the examination on clinical pathology and criminology, and I feel comfortable about my grade. Later on I learn that Dr. Kim says that you have German measles.

§ § §

In Korea, in the latter part of February, winter goes off and spring comes on. For this reason, the commencement ceremony of Chonnam University's Class of 1963, which includes the Medical

School, is held outdoors at Yong Bong University Square (the Dragon Phoenix Square). The square is crammed with a thousand graduates who are surrounded by throngs of relatives and friends. During the ceremonies, unexpectedly, a heavy snow like a silent blessing showers down on the square and over all the graduates, faculty members, and guests. They stand still and receive the heavenly benediction. The wind is laid asleep; the air is soft; in a brief period, the pouring flakes whiten the square and all the people on it because each snowflake is unusually large, like a petal of a white rose. Despite the thick snow, we graduates are able to receive our diplomas without getting a good drenching; rather we delight in the unforgettable memory of pouring spring snow.

Hyun A, as our ceremony is over—still the snow is sifting down—you and your daddy and the whole group of our family are awaiting my coming. You bring a bunch of red roses tied with red ribbon; as you hand it into my arms to congratulate me on my graduation, all the family behind you clap for you and me and laugh joyously. Your uncles, your aunts, and your cousins are there; your daddy's friend, Professor Oh Gook Choo, the Chairman of the Physics Department of Chonnam University, takes a picture of the three of us—Daddy, you, and me—in the snow at the crowded square. You are six years old; you have your two hands in your pockets, and you crouch against the heavy snow and the cold air. The snowflakes are piling up on the shoulders of your little red coat and the ribbons of your black hair. You look like Alice in Wonderland of the storybook. I feel proud of you to my very bones. And Hyun A, do you know, I fancy you holding a diploma, too, and wearing a black graduation cap with tangling tassels and a long black graduation gown with wide yellow lapels just like mine. I thank my family and friends for having made the long journey for today's celebration. Above all, I thank your daddy, the person who made possible my impossible dream.

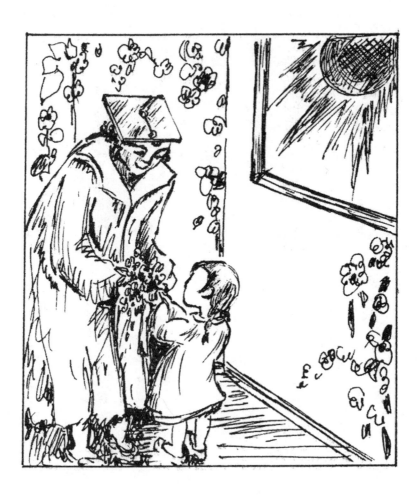

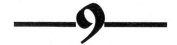

—9—

Beginning My Residency

Dear Hyun A,

In March 1963, I become a rotating intern in the Chonnam Medical School Hospital. In September of that year, the orthopedic department is my rotating turn. One afternoon I scrub up for the emergency case of a diabetic's left leg amputation.

The surgical hall is lined with scrubbing sinks, and the air is filled with the smell of Lysol. When I enter the operating room, Dr. Kim Hyung Soon and Dr. Yoon Jae Rong are already standing by the operating table. They wear sterile gloves and long, clean, white gowns, and their heads and mouths are covered with white cloth caps and thick gauze masks. They are brilliant young associate professors—stars in their profession. The circulating

nurse is prepping the patient's operating site with dark-brown iodine, and the scrub nurse in a sterile gown and gloves is arranging
the instruments and materials needed beside the operating table. The
circulating nurse covers the patient with a white cloth sterile sheet
and exposes the left lower thigh, and she adjusts the huge, bright,
pendant surgical lamp to focus on the operating site. The patient's x-
ray films are beside the anesthesiologist, who has put the patient to
sleep. My role will be to help the surgeons by holding retractors for
them, wiping blood to clear the operating field, and learning by watching and listening to their explanations.

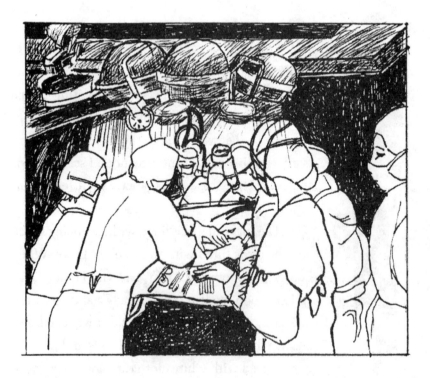

    Dr. Yoon holds the scalpel blade and measures and figures the
exact spot for the incision; with lighting speed he cuts down to the

bone. A large, glistening femur juts out from the bloody severed thigh muscles. Dr. Yoon then saws the decayed leg off from the healthy part of the thigh. As the leg thuds to the floor, I feel my heart drop with that dead leg. The circulating nurse puts the leg in a large steel basin on the gray-green marble floor. What a sight to behold! The patient must be tall, for the amputated leg is lengthy. The black, parched, skeletal leg with its protruding bony knee joint lies there like a rotten, smelly carcass; its long, thick, curved, pale tonenails are fastened on that decayed foot like the claws of a leopard. It gives me nausea. I try to avert my eyes from it.

"Are you all right?" Dr. Yoon asks.

"You are not used to seeing such cases," Dr. Kim sympathizes with me.

"I am fine, thank you," I reply with self-possession.

But they are uneasy; they watch me closely. My maternity clothing is unable to cover up the eight-month pregnancy.

I am grateful for the opportunity to participate in this operation. It gives me an awareness of the responsibility of the medical doctor. To save this patient's life, the surgeons had to sever the patient's gangrenous leg. I believe that they feel sorry for the patient—he lost part of his leg—but I also know that he gained his life because of the skill of these doctors. Only their conviction of their professional duty to the patient's health allows them to do such a repugnant thing. They overcame a disgusting and difficult situation; if I wish to be a medical doctor, I must follow in their footsteps.

In the future, as a medical doctor, I will do things more repulsive than today's case to save human lives. Although I am greatly shocked by this amputation surgery, I command myself to keep my mind straight—not to faint or to withdraw from the operating room. Only one thought—my professional duty to save patients' lives as other doctors do——makes me finish that case with Dr. Kim and Dr. Yoon.

Throughout the surgery my baby is kicking around and playing, not knowing what I am seeing and doing and thinking.

§   §   §

In the course of my internship, on November 14, 1963, your younger brother Steve is born at Gae Rim Dong in your maternal grandmother's house and is breast fed for eight months. After completion of a one-year program of internship, I am accepted by the Department of OB and Gyn of Chonnam University Medical Hospital——the same hospital in which I have an internship——as a resident in the four-year program.

The field of specialty is already decided before an internship starts. To enter a specific field requires many considerations, because once the field is declared, that field is decided for all one's professional lifetime. As I move through my final years of medical school, I try to determine which field most interests me, and I ask advice from the staff of each department. Every opinion suggests that I must select the field that I am most interested in, disregarding both current trends and financial gain. So I unroll my lists and draw my final conclusions.

First, I like to do surgery. It gives me satisfaction, since open tissue allows me to see clearly what is wrong and accordingly to fix the problem. The patient's recovery is prompt, and often surgery eradicates problems immediately, eliminating guessing games with laboratory data, equivocal symptoms, and the administrations of medicines. Second, I feel far more comfortable handling female patients than males. Third, I would like to keep up in all fields of medicine, if possible, not ignoring areas such as internal medicine, pediatrics, pathology, and endocrinology.

I think my way through these facts: If I pick the field of surgery, I must include male patients in my care. If I choose internal medicine, I will be discontented because I will have to borrow many indirect diagnostic tools, Besides, the course of recovery in internal medicine is so long and sometimes ends without improvement. Too, I would have to deal with male patients—not that I dislike or reject men, but I am not accustomed to caring for them. Hyun A, I know that you will say, petulantly, "Mom, you are so picky and trivial! A doctor's profession is a mission; whether you like it or not, a doctor must treat all patients, regardless of their gender!" But this is *my* choice.

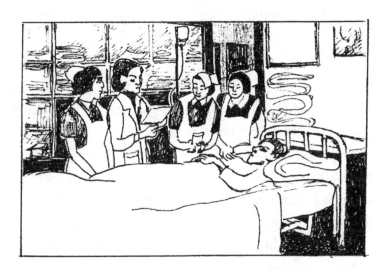

I think further, what if I become a pathologist? I am less interested in dealing with morgues than with the living; I cannot expect miracles from dead bodies. Then I think, how about being a pediatrician? But if I rotate to the Department of Pediatrics, I find at the office that there is always a baby with one of his parents or one of his family so that the room is crowded and noisy. Moreover, babies and children cannot give their exact complaints; instead, mothers or attendants give information about their sicknesses. And they seem so fragile and delicate. I do not think I can be a pediatrician.

Although becoming an obstetrician requires long hours of work, especially in the night, I decide to be an obstetrician and gynecologist. I will have surgery; I will see and treat female patients only; I will keep up a balanced medical knowledge in pathology, endocrinology, internal medicine, pediatrics, and surgery. Best of all, only in this field does the doctor manage two lives at the same time—mother and baby. This is the happiest field of medicine because it deals with the creation of life. Unlike the departments that care for old, incurable, gloomy and depressed patients, doctors in obstetrics and gynecology see brighter, younger, happier, and healthier patients. This field, OB and Gyn, will be my calling for the rest of my life.

§   §   §

Now I am a first-year resident in the OB & Gyn Department of Chonnam Medical School Hospital, and I will stay here for four more years until I complete my residency program. Therefore, prior to Steve's birth, we must move into another house that is within five minutes' walking distance from the hospital where I work. The reason is primarily that I plan to nurse Steve, and, secondly, I want to accommodate my working circumstances to our family life. At times your dad and I feel like migrating birds that follow the change of seasons since we so often have to move our shelters here and there.

In our OB & Gyn. Department there are three main faculty members: Professors Moon Byung Kap, Lee Sang Gun, and our chairman, Professor Kim Doo Sang. My first year of residency is exceptionally challenging. Usually each new residency has two members, but in our first year we have the exceptional number of seven residents. This is because five of them have been discharged from military service. These men are older and are very intent on a superb performance, and they bring up the level of the entire group. We all work so hard—I especially, for I am the only woman in the group.

Our chairman, Professor Doo Sang Kim, is a well-known authority in the field of the surgical treatment of cervical cancer, not only in Korea but in the world. His articles have been printed in the *Novack Pathology Obstetrics & Gynecology Textbook.* After he trained in West Germany, he worked in the West German Hospital in Pusan, Korea. He is an aspiring scholar and surgeon, and a devoted professor and medical doctor. Through his ardent passion for his profession, all his patients, medical students, and residents benefit fully. Because of his broad interests in many areas—especially in pathology, endocrinology, and infertility—a Papanicolaou cytology lab has been set up in our department for the first time, and we residents all stain specimen slides and read them by ourselves. In addition, pathological tissue slides are reviewed at our department. Regularly, at the weekly journal meetings, we residents review the *American Journal of Obstetrics & Gynecology.* We constantly prepare reviews of difficult cases to present, and we have to review many books and materials.

No residents have time for fooling around if they are to keep up with Professor Doo Sang Kim. By virtue of his rigorous training, at the end of our fourth year, all of us residents pass our OB & Gyn. Board Examination with distinguished scores, and every one of us has confidence in his own skill and knowledge to open his own medical practice. I can still picture Professor Kim as he walks: his paces are so fast and light that his upper body inclines forward as though a flying white busy bee is wearing a doctor's gown. He is always busy. His air is gentle, tidy, and noble; and when he smiles his gentle smile, he closes his shrewd eyes. With great respect and affection, we all cherish our special time with him.

§   §   §

One day in 1964 in late spring, I stroll during my lunch hour up a flight of steps to the medical school library, which is perched on the hilltop. Before entering the library, I stop to take a deep breath of the spring air. I am somewhat puffed up because Dr. Kim said to me that tonight, on call, I have permission to deliver babies by myself. Standing here, I look down at the hospital terrain and beyond. I see the busy street that runs along the west wall of the hospital. At the end of the wall, by the street, a small police station guards the populated area.

On the hill and the ground, all life pulses with spring; spring is graduating into early summer. Within the wall, under the leaden sky, the pale pink blossoms cluster so thickly on the twigs of the cherry trees that every bough is invisible, and the trees seem to be giant flowers. White and crimson wide-open petals cling to the bare dogwood branches like resting butterflies; deep-pink tiny blossoms cling to the leafless branches of the pinkbud trees. New maple leaves, light green or dark red, shadow the hilltop library.

And now in the early evening, a twenty-five-year-old patient comes to the delivery room in active labor. This is her first pregnancy, and her due date has already passed by two days. The whole course of her pregnancy has been uneventful without any complication. She is five feet tall and slender; her bulging abdomen looks bigger than she herself. I do a vaginal examination; her cervix already is opened half way, and the baby's head is down to the bottom of the pelvis. Her vital signs are normal. After giving routine orders to the oncall nurse, I am a little tense but even more excited, thinking of delivering a baby by myself. But I am weary from the long hours of working, and just for a moment I go to the verandah of the second story, lean against the white rail, and gaze up toward heaven. Dusk is gathering swiftly; the small, silvery full moon is veiled by gauzy gray mists on the southeast sky, drawing a red-orange circle around her. Despite the gloomy sky, the air is nearly perfect: not stuffy, not sultry—not even a breeze puffs by—but it is pleasant, soft, and calm. It could hold me all night in its bosom.

On my way back to the oncall room, I stop by my patient's room. The fierce labor pains assail her exactly and regularly like a machine; they come automatically every two or three minutes, lasting for a minute. The intensity of the pain becomes incremental. Her husband sits in a chair; he does not know what to do. Her mother-in-law supports her back, wiping her brow with a towel, and her sister-in-law dampens her parched lips with a wet cloth. At every pain, the girl is subjected to torment. She is pleading to her mother-in-law, "Aigo, Baeya! [This insufferable pain!] I am dying, mother!" She looks exhausted, having sunken sleepy eyes, dry, flaky lips, and pale depressed cheeks. Her slender arms and legs seem no longer able to bear that pain. I ask her if she wants any pain medication. She refuses it for the sake of the baby's safety. "Why don't you get a little shot to take the edge off your pain?"

"No, no..." replies she. And she writhes in agony. "Aigo Baeya! Aigo Baeya! I am dying, mother!"

Such a little and fragile patient but with a mighty heart for her baby. I check the baby's heartbeats, which are strong and regular. Before leaving the room, I hear again her desperate entreating, "Aigo, Umma [Oh momma!] I can take this no more!"

"Ay Myunura [Oh, my daughter-in-law!] your doctor said your pain won't be long! Bear it just a little more!" her mother-in-law soothes her, wiping her drenched brow and eyes.

In the oncall room, Dr. Song, the senior resident, gives me important tips: how I should protect the perineum from tearing, how, as soon as the baby's head is out, I should wipe the baby's mouth clean of amniotic fluid; how and where I should clamp the cord and cut between the two clamps. I review the labor and delivery section from Williams' textbook and actually practice the delivery process with a model of a fetus and pelvis and birth canal. Then I fall asleep.

Just past midnight, I can hear distant thunder rumbling, brewing a storm and breaking the silence of the night; it has no end but bubbles faintly like a simmering hot spring. A soft swish of wind brings raindrops to tap the window panes gently; soon afterward, I hear a slender stream murmur down into the hollow gutter. Suddenly a streak of lightning flashes at the window, and the thunder vibrates in the dark void as if thousands of ancient drums are beating at once and dwindling away into the same dark vacancy. Tonight's darkness does not bring rest and silence. Instead, tumultuous thunderbolts in heaven and a tormented mother in labor on the rainy earth create an extraordinary night.

After a while the nurse's phone call wakes me, and I examine my patient's progress. She is ready to deliver. She is transferred to the delivery room; the nurses put her into the delivery position, prep her with antiseptic iodine solution on the perineum and inner thighs, and drape her with sterile sheets and leg covers. I sit before her on the round portable chair, and I suddenly see the turbid membrane bulging out of the birth canal. It swiftly bursts, splashing my face, including my spectacles. The nurse takes off my glasses and wipes them clean. I feel my lower chest is wet too. When I see the tip of the baby's black hair, I become frantic and seem to forget everything that I have practiced, but I try to keep my wits about me. Once a baby is coming down through the birth canal, one strong push forces the baby right down on the perineum. The nurse and I ask the mother not to push down, instead, to open her mouth and blow out that pressure through her mouth so that the perineum can be protected. The baby smoothly slides out and in a second is crying in my hands. But my heart is pounding under my wet gown, for I was only a hair's breadth from dropping him to the marble delivery room floor. I had not realized that a baby is so slippery.

I clamp the cord and cut it correctly. But as I see the long, plump cord with the webs of convoluted blood vessels that connects the baby's belly with his mother, my fear flashes through and makes my hand tremble because I feel that I am going to cut off the life blood line. Yet to cut with my own hand the life bloodline of the umbilical cord is a great event. I realize that I have just helped to set free the perfect, independent, individual creature to the wide open world. For the first time I feel the pride of being a doctor and obstetrician. I lift the baby high toward the mother, saying, "Mrs. Jyung, here is your baby, look, a baby boy!"

The mother is crying, tears of genuine joy, "I cannot believe it! That is my baby!"

She is sniffing back her tears, exclaiming again, "O my baby! O my baby!" She eagerly tries to hold the baby, stretching out both her arms toward the baby. While I deliver the placenta and repair the perineum, the nurse swathes the baby and hands him to the mother. My patient is stable, so I hurry to the waiting room to give the family the good tidings. I see their anxious, worried eyes, but after hearing my report, they stand and shout with joy, huddling together.

I return to the oncall room exhausted. Notwithstanding my weariness, my heart swells with exhilaration; I cannot go to bed, so I draw open the curtains to the waning night. All is silent and lies sound asleep. All commotion in the heavens and in the delivery room is gone. The silvery streaks of dawn enlarge before my eyes into yellow orange beams, reflections of the universal light behind the dark horizon.

§   §   §

At last, the time comes to perform my first C-section. My patient is at full term in her first pregnancy and has had a long, difficult labor caused by the baby's abnormal position and her narrow pelvis. Before surgery, to make absolutely sure of the pelvic anatomy and the surgical procedures—albeit I know all that—I review the C-section from Williams' textbook. However, I am afraid. The closer the time comes to getting into the operating room, the faster and harder my heartbeats throb. Everything I reviewed seemed to be forgotten. But once I enter the operating room and see the patient on the table my thought flies: "If I don't take care of her right now, their lives—hers and her baby's—are in danger." Only that thought remains; other worries and fears vanish. Now I can concentrate on what I must do.

My supervisor, Professor San Gun Lee, and another senior resident, Dr. Kim, scrub with me. Every time I incise the patient's tissue, blood pours out and gets into the operating field. When I open the abdominal cavity, there is nothing in my view but a taut, glistening, gigantic uterus pushing up to the diaphragm. I incise further, opening the uterine muscle, and with my right hand scoop the baby's head out of the deep pelvic cavity. Quickly I wipe amniotic fluid from the baby's mouth and the baby girl cries and wriggles vigorously. At that moment, I would not trade that cry for any price. My special attention goes to cut the cord between two clamps, not outside of them, for that would bring grave danger for both mother and baby. I peel the afterbirth off the mother's womb with my open right palm like the peel of an orange. A flood of blood sweeps over the operating field; delivering a baby is impossible without the sight of blood. Behold, what a mighty power the uterine muscle has! Before my eyes, its two extreme states—stretched and contracted—are disclosed. Instantly, after the delivery of the baby and the placenta, it shrinks from the big ballooned state to the size of a football. It is rock solid, so only the surgical needle can pierce it through; I sew the uterus closed. I check the patient's other pelvic organs—tubes and ovaries—and count the instruments and sponges. Then I close her abdomen. The patient tolerates her surgery and will recover well.

After surgery, I realize that an abdominal delivery as compared to a vaginal delivery demands great speed of performance because it directly correlates with both the mother and the baby's danger and safety. But in both the abdominal and vaginal deliveries, the sight of a pool of blood is so scary!

Hyun A, do you know what I do this evening? After I see the patient and healthy newborn baby, I go to her family in the waiting room to congratulate them and inform them of the mother and baby's condition. My head and heart swell like a mighty river, for I have become a real obstetrician. I am overwhelmed by joy, confidence, and pride like a triumphant hero who returns from the battlefield after defeating a mortal enemy. It seems the whole world is mine. So I stop by the market to buy beef and tofu; to celebrate my first C-section with my family, I prepare a fine dinner for our family of four. I tell your daddy and you—of course, Steve is a little baby—all about how my adventure in the operating room went successfully today.

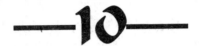

—10—

Steve's
Mysterious
Illness

Dear Hyun A,

In 1966, one fine October afternoon, our baby sitter comes to our department to tell me that the baby, Steve, has suddenly fallen ill. I rush home; I almost run for home. Steve has become pale and languid, lying on his bed; he refuses to eat, play, or babble. I strain freshly squeezed apple juice through gauze, which he used to drink. He refuses to drink even water.

Steve is almost two years old. He has been a perfectly healthy and happy baby. He has no fever, no diarrhea, no vomiting. Your daddy and I try everything, but nothing makes him better, so we take him to Dr. Chul Son, who is the head of the pediatric department in our hospital and whose reputation for healing children is well known in the town. Dr. Son diagnoses Steve's condition as an acute dehydration that requires Steve to be admitted to the hospital and to be given intravenous fluids. Dr. Son says that he will observe Steve closely. All kinds of blood tests and x-ray examinations fail to reveal the cause of Steve's illness. A bottle of 500 cc of Ringer's lactate solution plus multiple vitamins is connected to a long, transparent tube that goes into Steve's right arm.

Every day Dr. Son examines our baby, palpating his neck, opening his eyes, and ears, looking at his throat, listening to his lungs and heart with a stethoscope. He palpates his sunken abdomen and checks his knee reflexes by hitting the knee tendons with a red rubber hammer.

He asks us, "Has Steve ever been sick before?"

"No, he has been a perfectly healthy child," replies your dad. "In fact he never was still a moment except when he was asleep."

"The results of the blood tests and x-ray examinations do not show the course of his illness," Dr. Son says.

He is silent for a moment, that says to us, "So far I would do nothing other than what I have been doing." And he goes out of the room with a trail of residents to continue making his rounds.

Steve's condition keeps getting worse as his veins collapse. The doctors can hardly find a vein to give further intravenous fluid, so they have to open his right ankle vein by a procedure called a cutdown and with great difficulty insert a tube to supply the IV fluid. Dr. Son has tried everything possible for more than two weeks, but there is no hope of improvement, and Steve is dying. Dr. Son does not want the baby to die in the hospital, and your dad and I agree. So the doctor takes the tube out from Steve's cutdown vein. We wrap our baby in a blanket, and your daddy holds him. Your daddy and I and your Gae Rim Dong grandmother—my mother—leave the hospital lobby together. Your grandmother is almost beside herself at losing her grandson. She seems to be going mad in her grief. She begs us to go back to the old Korean cure of the herb doctor, screeching, "Steve will die either way—whether or not we take him to the herb doctor. But if we take him to her, even if he dies, we will have no regret that we left anything undone."

She knows that your daddy and I don't believe in the herb doctor's sham. But we agree without hesitation, since we are desperate to try anything for Steve before he dies. It appears to be a last resort. Instead of going home, we call a taxi and go directly from the gate of the hospital to the herb doctor's. No one speaks; we clench our hands into fists; on the way, the grandmother keeps peeking at Steve, opening the blanket; she wants to check that he is still breathing. We ride in the taxi in silence for an endless fifteen minutes.

The herb doctor's house is nestled amid the crowded city blocks. We meander as if we are in a maze, but we finally pull up to the small house with its blue-tiled roof. The small wooden gate faces to the south and is closed but not locked. A tall straw fence surrounds the house.

The little house is typical of that of a simple Korean family. We enter the gate and pass into the small, neatly swept yard. In front of the house is a long, knee-high wooden platform (*maru*) that measures four by twelve feet. Two pairs of rubber shoes—one pair for a man, the other for a woman—are set outside.

At the left corner of the yard stands a large tree laden with red persimmons. At the right side of the yard close to the fence are the following three items: first, a small flower bed with red and purple zinnias, pink garden balsams, and pink cosmos; next, a six by six raised concrete square for the ceramic pantry is open to the sun, with its various-sized black ceramic pots for storing soybean sauces and paste, hot paste, salted fish, and pickled vegetables; and finally, a well that is protected by a thigh-high concrete tube measuring four feet in diameter.

"Is anybody here? Is the herb doctor *Ajumma* (lady) here?" your grandmother calls anxiously. A middle-aged woman opens the door and walks out on the wooden platform. She is rather short and chubby and plain, and wears a white cotton *jugori* (top) and black cotton *chima* (long skirt) and *bosun* (cloth socks).

"Come please and sit on the maru," she greets us. "What's wrong?"

"Here, we brought my grandson. You should look at him right away and should do something for him. He is very, very sick." Your grandmother opens the blanket and shows her Steve. She just looks at him for a second—she does not even use her finger to touch or to examine him.

"Oh, oh, something is stuck in his stomach!" she murmurs to herself. She runs into her kitchen and brings out a white soup bowl. Then she runs to the well, seizing the straw rope and drawing up fresh water in a wooden bucket. She washes her hands at the well and pours fresh water into the bowl and sets it on the maru.

She has your grandmother hold Steve firmly. She massages Steve's stomach all over as if she is searching for something, and then takes hold of something. She pushes the thing up to the base of the esophagus. Still holding the thing with her left hand, she dips her ugly, knobbed index and middle fingers into the white bowl. She swiftly puts her two fingers into Steve's small mouth and deep down into his throat, so that the left hand and the right hand meet, and the thing that she found at the stomach is shoved up into Steve's throat to meet her two fingers. In a blink she takes her fingers out of Steve's mouth and shows us a swollen brown-gray seed of a persimmon.

"This was stuck and imbedded in his stomach. Otherwise, there is nothing wrong with him. He will be all right now."

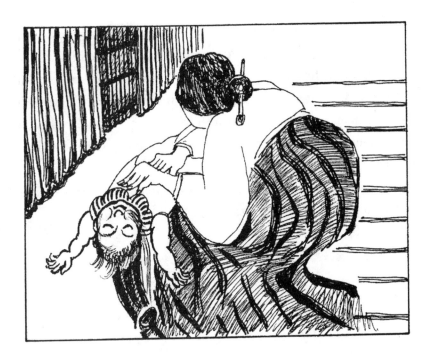

We look at the seed. It is exactly like those of the persimmons we had eaten the evening before Steve started to be sick. Our uncle, who lived in our home town, had brought a basketful of large and well-ripened persimmons as his gift. We had eaten a few of them; the rest of them were put on the desk that was not high enough to be out of Steve's reach. He must have pulled down and eaten a persimmon and swallowed the seed. If we had put the persimmon basket on a high shelf, we would have avoided this disaster.

It is unbelievable that the minute she takes out the seed, we hear Steve heave a deep sigh; we can see the pallor of his little face change into a glow as though we are watching the breaking dawn in the eastern sky. We try to give him water; for the first time since his sickness, he touches the water cup.

"Give him liquid first, then gradually add solid food," the herb doctor advises.

"Now my cub is revived! His life is returned!" your grandmother cries in raving joy. "Ajumma, I cannot thank you enough!"

On the way home, Steve wriggles in your daddy's arms, looking out the window. At home, grandmother makes boiled rice water; he drinks a cup and gets up and plays. Since then, this illness has become Steve's anecdote: "Grandmother saved Steve's life when he almost died from a persimmon seed."

It is sheer miracle. A miracle must remain unexplained. If explained, it would not be a miracle.

—11—

Completing the Residency

Dear Hyun A,

Now I am a third-year resident, and my special knowledge and surgical technique and clinical attitude and wisdom about handling patients begin to give me real confidence. I feel more and more sure about what I am doing, which gives me enthusiasm as well as interest in my work. Your dad holds the position of Chairman of the Department of Physics at Chosun University; he loves what he teaches. Steve has never been sick since that mysterious illness. Your youngest brother, Robert, is over four months old. You are in the third grade at Susack Elementary School.

In the summer of that year, as part of the hospital residency program, I am assigned for three months to be trained at the Missionary Jae Jung

Hospital, which is located at the outskirts of Kwangju City. People call this city "Midori Oka," which means—the term is Japanese—"the green hill." This vast and exclusive territory—idyllic, serene, and peaceful—is private property that belongs to the Christian mission. The high hills are covered with lush, thick woods, the best scenic view in the city. The high stories of western style large white houses for the missionaries are nestled and wrapped by greenery. Occasionally, a few of the missionaries' little children roll down the hills on their bikes. The girls among them put white flower baskets on the front of their bikes. Their golden hair shines under the bright sun; their fair skin, blue eyes, and plump, well-nourished little bodies all suggest little angels in the garden to me, for at that time we had never been exposed to people from other continents like Europe or America or Africa.

Among these hills, the renowned Speer Girls Junior and High School was founded by a missionary, Miss Speer. The principal of the school is still an American missionary, but the rest of the teachers are all Koreans. This school has trained many great woman leaders and pioneers of organizations such as the YWCA and the Sung Bin Yeu Sook (Sacred Poverty Institution) for the enlightenment of women's education and modernization. One of the most prominent persons in this movement was Cho A Ra. In this missionary terrain, above the girls' school and the missionary residencies, the huge two-story Jae Jung Hospital rises above the green trees.

Jae Jung Hospital is a charitable hospital established and operated by the Presbyterian Christian Missionary Charitable Organization. This is a general hospital with many important departments: internal medicine, pediatrics, surgery, obstetrics and gynecology, anesthesiology. However, at this time, tuberculosis is an epidemic. This hospital is like a sanitarium and plays the very important role of preventing and treating the ill, both medically and surgically. Every day a flood of sickly, poor patients crowds the hospital as inpatients and outpatients.

Inside, the hospital is always mopped clean and is well organized. The director, Dr. Ronald Dietrick, besides his important administrative job, does his duty as a surgeon. He possesses unlimited energy for work, is very frugal, very wise, and skillfully manages the hospital both medically and financially without wasting a penny. All the doctors and nurses are devoted and compassionate and are efficient in their work. They are all different from the people outside this hospital and are steeped in their religious belief. The Being above us seems to form their second nature. This hospital deserves its fine reputation.

Even though the OB-Gyn department of the hospital is small in scale, I still deliver babies either vaginally or abdominally and do other gynecological surgeries as I did at our medical school hospital. I have to add certain things such as special instruments for our surgeries and new necessary programs for the department. For the outpatients, the hospital has an enormous number of samples of vaginal creams and birth control pills. In Korea at this time these medicines are not generally available. These samples make my work easier and at the same time make the patients happier.

One summer afternoon, the hospital staff go to attend a funeral ceremony at the chapel in Midori Oka, the Missionary Hill. The seven-year-old son of Missionary Smith has drowned. The small ceremony is held in the little chapel. The atmosphere is very quiet, very reserved.

"Look, look at Mrs. Smith! She does not cry!" someone whispers behind me. "She believes her son Tom is in heaven with Jesus Christ; she can see him there."

Throughout the funeral service, no one cries. The chapel is peaceful and tranquil. Mrs. Smith keeps her calm composure; she tries to console her guests. If a Korean mother had lost a child, she would not hold in her sorrow but would have burst into loud weeping, whether in public or in private. She would have thought her son's death was the last time to see him. How different is behavior when it comes from different thinking! Men who have religious faith in God surrender themselves to God and transcend to a higher realm than men usually inhabit.

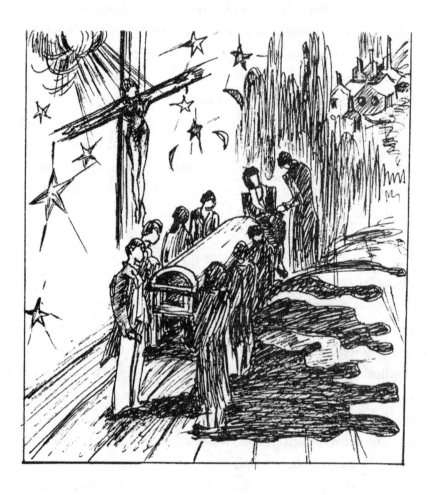

In connection with transcendence, around the end of my three-month rotation program, I question myself about one particular doctor. Dr. H. Cogington, an American, is head of internal medicine and the former hospital administrator. Why, I ask, does he have to go through all these tribulations? If he wanted to avoid them, he could live comfortably in his own rich country. He is the first doctor every morning to come to the hospital to work. He is the last doctor to leave the hospital at night. Why, in this poor and underdeveloped foreign country, has he exposed himself to the dangerous environment of tuberculosis and other terrible diseases and taken this burden on himself and on his family? Yet no matter how sick, or how dirty, or how poor his patients are, he, with his compassion, treats them kindly. He tries hard to communicate with his patients, using the Korean language and keeping his Korean dictionary in his pocket. Finally, I answer myself, "Without the love of God in him, he could never have given himself to such an extreme degree to work for the disadvantaged." I feel he is a saint on earth. And the people in Jae Jung Hospital call him "Jesus."

§   §   §

And now one more year has rolled away from us. You are a fourth grader; you have grown taller, prettier, and smarter. Your private tutor, Aunt Sun Hi, a senior high school student, comes to our home five days a week from Monday to Friday. At home your daddy hangs up a blackboard on the wall of the front porch for your tutoring hours. At school you are at the top of your class and a monitor for your class. After your homework and tutoring hours end, you bring your friends from our village; you all play in our yard: jumprope, hopscotch, softball. Most of all, you sing songs together—alone, by turn, in rounds, or in a chorus. The echoes of singing and playing

resound all over our village. For this reason, the villagers call our
house a school; for this is new to Korean tradition.

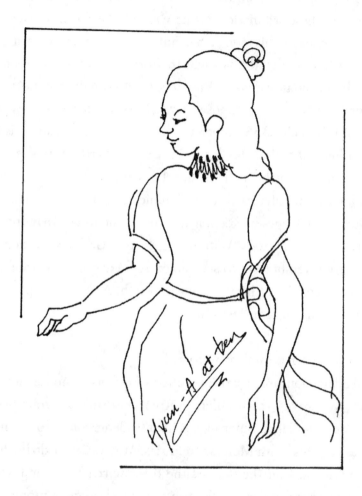

One evening I come home late from the hospital. I feel guilty
for neglecting my children. "I am so sorry I couldn't come home
early; an emergency case arrived. Your friends' mothers take good
care of your friends, but I cannot give the same care to you and your

brothers," I say to you. Do you know how your immediate answer surprises me?

"I like my mother more than my friends' mothers because they only take care of their children but *my* mother takes care of many, many sick patients and delivers babies at the same time that she takes care of my brothers and me."

When my ten-year-old daughter says this to me, at first I cannot believe my ears. You already have the foundation of the philosophy of advanced human behavior. I only regret that no one is there to hear what you said to me!

My duties escalate, with longer working hours, more responsibility for the patients' care, more materials to read and memorize. Most of all, I have a family, three children to take care of. Even though your daddy and you are exceedingly independent of me—rather, you both try to help me—my obligation to my family never decreases. And now I come to the last year of training, and I must take the OB-Gyn Board Examination. My years of commitment are put to the test. In early summer, after riding a train for more than fourteen hours, we seven residents go to Seoul for the examination. We have all worked so hard. And we all pass.

Without a break, your daddy decides to go to America for further study; I am to go with him. The AMA (American Medical Doctors Association) requires the certification that can be acquired only after passing the ECMFG (Examination for College of Medicine Foreign Graduate), both written and oral. In the late fall, I ride a train again to Seoul for the examination. I miraculously survive a volley of tests. Immediately I apply to American hospitals and am accepted by St. Vincent Hospital, Toledo, Ohio. Your daddy and I decide to fly to America.

—12—

Flight to the
New Land

Dear Hyun A,

Man's life is a journey, an adventure to whatever man desires to be or to have. Because of man's desire to explore space, Neil Armstrong rode a spacecraft on July 20, 1969, and landed on the moon. With the same drive of human spirit, your daddy and I rode an airplane, which carried us to America on June 20, 1969.

Once the airplane lifts off the ground and folds three rolling wheels to its bosom, our familiar world is utterly separated and left behind us. The further the plane flies, the further we are from that world; on the other hand, we grow closer to the strange world. The people surrounding us on the plane look strange: they are tall, with white skin, blond hair, and blue eyes; the clothing they wear and the food they give us to eat and the gestures they use are different from ours; the language that they speak is entirely alien to our ears; even the written letters look strange. But we have no alternative; we are forced to speak English to communicate with our fellow travelers.

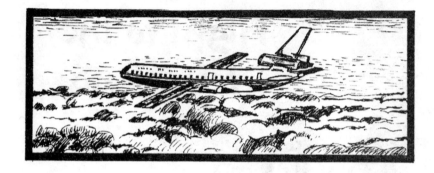

I am abruptly thrown into an unfamiliar world. I am curious about it; at the same time I feel anxious about plunging into the new world as an alien. Despite my curiosity and apprehension, when I look at the space through the plane's small oval window, the blue sky is the same familiar sky; when I look down on the silvery blue Pacific Ocean, the familiar blue face of the boundless water comforts me.

I listen to the stewardesses' announcements and questions, to the captain's welcome and weather report, and to the other passengers' conversation, and I can grasp only partial meaning of their speaking. My confidence in my schoolroom English grows shaky, and I become tense and apprehensive as we approach our destination. For I have an important job to perform—to see, to hear, to diagnose, and to treat the sick—just as native English-speaking medical doctors do, in spite of my language barrier. The disquiet and anxiety I feel now is somewhat different from my uneasiness at leaving my homeland. Now I feel the restlessness and anxiety that comes before a battle begins: what if I am unable to understand my patients' complaints correctly? What if my patients are unable to understand my speech, my inquiries? What should I do to make our communication work? I sit and plan: I will attempt to convey my intentions and to understand their complaints by drawing pictures, by making sounds, and by using body language. Then, my communication among patients and doctors and nurses should improve daily. As the airplane flies through the sky from Seoul, Korea, to Tokyo, Japan, to Seattle, Washington, so my brain works uninterruptedly through the long hours.

An English-speaking woman in her thirties sits beside me. She is tall, plump, and blond; her fair complexion needs no make up; she has large blue eyes and red lips. Everything that she has looks big. She wears a vibrant red-blue flowered dress, which is becoming to her. She talks with her husband and reads a magazine which has women's pictures on it. When the stewardess starts distributing lunch, the woman asks me, "Where are you going?"

"I—I—I go to Toledo Ohio," I haltingly answer.

"Why are you going to America?" She slows her speed of speaking and pronounces every word clearly.

"M—m—m I am a medical doctor and I like to learn the advanced medical techniques." I try to pronounce the words correctly, but it goes awkwardly.

"Is this the first time to go to America?" She seems to sympathize with my poor English.

"Yes, this is my first time to America." I brace myself to speak English with her and continue:

"I am going to St. Vincent Hospital Toledo, Ohio, for the residency program. My name is Chi Sun Yoo. I married and I have three children: one daughter and two sons. My daughter is eleven years old; my elder son is m-m five years old; my younger son, our baby son, is two years old. They m-m-m are at home in Korea."

I mumble but she seems to understand me. "Who is taking care of your children?" she expresses some kind of motherly compassion.
"With my mother," I reply with an assured tone.
"Oh good! That's good!"
And she shows me how to put butter on a roll and how to cut a piece of ham using a fork and knife. The buttered bread is so soft and tasty; bacon strips and scrambled eggs and frosted cake are so delicious. Everything is oily and sweet and bland in contrast to Korean red-hot, salty, spicy foods. I eat everything on my tray. Then she starts to talk about her name and her status. I cannot understand everything, but I glean some from her because she uses easy words, speaks slowly, and pronounces the words clearly.

She is thirty-three years old and has been married for ten years without children, though she has been trying. So she is going to receive an adopted child, a girl three years old, from Korea in three months. She has already furnished the baby's room, and she has the baby's clothes. She and her husband went on a trip to Korea one week ago. They visited her brother-in-law in the United States Army. They could not see their adopted daughter, who is now in one of the orphanages in Korea, because all laws are subject to the adoption agency's rules where all information is closed except for the child's pictures and the child's physical examination report. They enjoyed their trip to Korea: the people, the country, and the customs. They live in New York City. Her husband is a professor of biology.

Her companionship makes my journey easier and lighter. It is my first flight, and it is inconceivable that I should fly thirty-five thousand feet high above the clouds. Nothing is above us but the blazing sun in the blue void. Nothing is below us but layers and layers of white clouds, creating a white cloud ocean that is pendant in the vacant, boundless space. Even though the plane flies without pause and more than 460 miles an hour, I feel we all are still. When the sun hides from us, darkening over the cloud ocean and its hem of horizon, I have never seen such dreadful depth of darkness, as though we are sinking into a cosmic black hole. The first sleep in the night sky is not much different than that on earth: there a sleep brings me dreams and restoration of vigor. The dream took me home; two boys, Kwan Woong and Young Shik, are, as usual, playing with dirt in front of our gate, waiting for me to come home from work about 5:30 p.m. They see me and they are running toward me, calling, "Yumma!" [Mamma]. I open my arms to hug them. Then the dream is gone, leaving me in the plane seat. What a mischief! Such dreams pierce men's sore hearts.

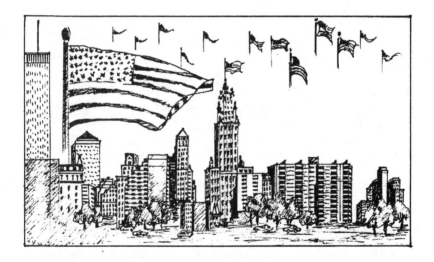

And now we arrive! My curiosity and excitement flame vehemently in my small heart. Everything around the airport's corridor looks grand, clean, and orderly. On the way to the main station from the terminal, three little girls are walking beside their mother. They seem to be eleven, ten, and nine and are walking barefoot on the corridor floor that is made of green-gray marble; its surface is smooth, clean, and shining like a Korean's living room floor; there is no litter strewn nor even visible dust. The children do not carry their shoes in their hands. They look so comfortable and utterly safe as they walk barefoot.

Curiously enough, even though such a multitude of people are steadily coming and going, no one has smudged mud or dirt on the floor. I notice that the Americans waiting are very taciturn and well-behaved; they sit, read, knit, or crochet, not disturbing others. They form orderly lines at boarding time. A Korean station is filled with shouts of welcome, with running children with laughter and tears at the time of departing and returning. On the contrary, here people are quiet and well-oriented to rules and regulations. They do not talk but seem autonomous, self-contained, and very, very private.

At Seattle, before my plane leaves for Chicago, your daddy has to catch another plane to go to Vancouver and on to Grand Fork, North Dakota. A woman clerk at the boarding counter directs him to go west toward the gates; my gate is to the north. We have no time to linger over our first separation in thirteen years of marriage. Our departure cleaves us into two. His last words were:

> "If you are uncertain about how to get to the gate for Chicago, you must again ask any officers or airline people. Remember, the rocket of our adventure has been already launched into space; we cannot get it back. We have to fight with whatever we have for our own and our children's futures. I will write and call you whenever I can. Good luck to you! Good-bye!"

He says this composedly, turns his back, joins the crowd, and marches on. I stand fixed and accept his leaving with resignation, eyeing his back moving off, wishing him a safe journey. What an evil Fate! She detaches three little children from us, leaving them behind in the faraway homeland; now here, on utterly alien soil, she snatches my husband away from me amidst a multitude of strangers, leaving me alone! I am as battered in my mind as though a shipwreck has left me on a far strand; I feel that I have just lost my mighty ship and the last ship's company. But there is no use crying over the loss of them.

I go to my gate. I see that here people look energetic, lively, cheerful and free; they walk fast; they use many body gestures with their conversation; they wear differently designed and colorful clothes. The women here do not look passive and shy; they look as active and courageous as men. Modesty and bashfulness do not appear to be women's virtues here. I walk on with the crowd toward the north gates. The long, wide way of the corridor bustles with the stream of people coming and going: among them a uniformed pilot and two stewardesses wheel their baggage; one father saddles his baby son on his neck; a mother puts her baby in a stroller; another father saddles his infant to his bosom in the baby sack, which is suspended from his shoulders (in Korea, only a mother carries the baby, tying the baby to her back with a long, wide cloth). Bright advertising pictures of the large hotels and airlines are hung on the walls of the corridors. All the people follow the signs and letters written for directions, gates, flights, departures, and arrivals. Vending machines for snacks and drinks stand here and there. It seems signs, letters, and machines regulate the order of the multitudes. I stop many times to ask people about how to reach my gate. Their smiles and kind directions become my strength.

I safely get into my plane seat to fly from Seattle to Chicago. Without my husband beside me, I feel crippled; I have lost my right wing. For the first time I am really alone in the strange, stark country. That notion alone stirs my anxiety, yet to see the vast land in all its strangeness exhilarates me.

A young man who looks like a college student sits at my right side; at my left sits a middle-aged woman who appears to be a teacher. This time I can pick up more of the words of the stewardess' directions. The woman next to me appears exhausted and falls into deep slumber until the stewardess brings her meal; the young man at my right is intensely preoccupied with reading. Then the meal forces him to give up his reading and to pay attention to his surroundings. "Where are you coming from?" he asks me.

"I am from Korea."

"Is this for a tour, or visiting, or immigration?"

"I——I——I am coming for medical training. I am hi——hired by St. Vincent Hospital in Toledo, Ohio." I am encouraged to practice my English. "What do you read?" I ask him.

"*Crime and Punishment,*"he replies, showing me the paperback's cover. "I am half-way through. This is my second time reading it," says he. "My name is Randy Johnston. I am a junior at the University of Chicago; my major is mathematics."

I ask him that if he has read half way through, he may have read that Raskolnikov said that to the real ruler, like Napoleon, "Everything is permitted; I killed not a human being but a principle."

"O, then, you have read this book!" He is trying to talk slowly with more body signs.

"Yes, I read the book in Korean language but not in English m-m when I was in junior high school and m——m sophomore college." I too express my fascination with the book. He asks me why I read it twice. I pause, thinking how to convey to him my love for this complicated and intriguing book with my stammering English. However, this is a good chance to practice English conversation so long as he permits me to talk. I will say to him as briefly as possible that this entire book——not just a part of it——is the highest psychoanalytic book. I try to give him my interpretation.

"I really admire Dostoevsky, who embodied the Christian spirit through the character of the prostitute," says the young man.

My body feels confused because of coming from east to west: at night I am wide awake, during the daytime, sleepy. So I fall asleep like the lady next to me. Already our plane has sped about six hours from Seattle. A stewardess is announcing that our plane is approaching O'Hare Airport in Chicago. The plane is swooping down through thick clouds, hurting my ears. Soon after, the plane's oval door opens to the vast masses of human dwellings which are veiled by hazy blue polluted air. The plane touches the ground with roars of glad grows and slowly rolls to the terminal!

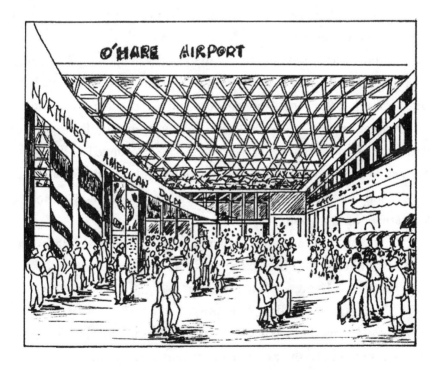

Ah, this is the second-largest city in America! This is America, the most advanced and largest and richest country in the world! Look at that vast landing ground, where numerous giant planes are departing and landing like white mammoth birds. Huge buildings surround the airport. Countless airplanes are perched to rest at the different terminals. The airport seems to be a city in itself.

The countless terminals cluster together, each with its own waiting station. Everywhere I look inside the buildings—in the terminals, corridors, and main stations—I see floods of people. Besides Caucasians, I see Blacks, Asians, turbaned and sari-wearing Arabs and Indians. People of each race look alike within their own race; I can hardly distinguish them. My head is spinning because I have more foreign signs, more written letters and machines to follow to reach my destination on time. I feel as if I am in a labyrinth. But by using all my five senses, I manage to get through the maze and reach the right flight to go to Detroit.

After an hour's flight, our plane arrives at Detroit Airport at 8:00 p.m. All the people who get off the plane go to the lower level to pick up their luggage. Here again the power of the machine under the control of men is exercised for the convenience of men. All of the bags—not one is alike, as every man's countenance is different—are riding on the steel rails, circling round and round until no baggage is left. At the custom office platform, there are many outlets to check everyone's passport and bags.

"Did you bring any food or plants, or drugs?" an officer asks me.

"No, but I—I—I have clothes and books."

"How much money did you bring?"

"Two thousand dollars."

He opens wide my two big bags and rummages through them and sends me out of the gate after stamping the date on my passport. There, a young man in a navy suit and red tie holds up a big card on which is written my name and St. Vincent Hospital, Toledo, Ohio. He greets me with a glad expression when he finds me and introduces himself by name, saying he has come from the Education Department of St. Vincent Hospital to pick me up. What a kind emissary from Heaven! He carries my bags to the front of the station and has me wait there. As soon as he pulls his car before me and puts the bags in his trunk, we leave for Toledo as the red sunset illuminates the back of our car. As we move closer to Toledo, the dusk grows thicker and a myriad of lights start to twinkle in the city, my first home in America.

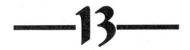

We Become
Americans

Dear Hyun A,

Now I come from the Oriental to the Occidental world completely alone to a different continent, America, which seems as fictitious as an overnight dream. In 1969, on the first of July, my internship starts at St. Vincent Hospital and Medical Center in Toledo, Ohio. The hospital has more than six hundred inpatient beds and is the biggest hospital in the city. Its medical educational program is well known as excellent for breadth of coverage, for warm, compassionate care, and for fine financial support and good living conditions for the medical trainees. In that year, the total number of interns is eight. We come from all over the world: Korea, the Philippines, Indonesia, Thailand, India, and America. I am the only woman, and the oldest. Our living quarters are shared with St. Vincent School of Nursing, which is located right by the main hospital building and so is convenient to our work both day and night.

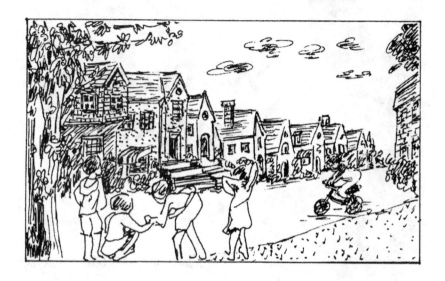

Most alien to me is not the land, not the people, not the customs, but *language,* the barrier of language. I feel as if someone has suddenly come and tied my tongue. I cannot talk as I want. The situation of helplessness reminds me that language is the basic and essential tool to communicate in any civilization. Therefore, for anyone who wants to live in a foreign country, the first and foremost thing to do is to learn the language that people in that land speak and write. At this initial stage, when I am taking the patients' histories, I face great difficulty in that the patients are no more able to understand me than I am able to understand what they are saying. This is because although I learned English grammar and read medical books throughout high school, medical college, and training periods, all of my English teachers were Koreans whose pronunciation and intonation were quite different from those of Americans. For instance, when I ask,

"Did you see bleeding?" I mean to ask about blood, but my patients understand me to say "breeding." So I write or spell out the word "bleeding." Sometimes I need to draw pictures to make them understand me. The kind nurses bridge over my quandaries many, many times.

During working time, like a sentinel over the midnight battle, I must be alert to every move about what I say, hear, watch, and do. My nerves and brain are utterly exhausted at the end of every day. Imagine, Hyun A, whoever comes to live in America without any education in the English language, what a hard time he would go through! He would think Americans are discriminating against him because he can't speak English, but that wouldn't be the whole truth. He may be discriminating against the Americans who cannot understand him. And if we had not learned any language besides our own tongue in childhood, to master another language in adulthood would prove terribly difficult.

Do you know what happens to me, Hyun A? The forced circumstance—nothing remains but to speak English—disallows me from speaking Korean, with no alternative, and this helps my progress in communicating more easily not only with patients but with attending physicians and the hospital staff. Attending physicians are accustomed to doctors coming from foreign lands who have language problems. They try to talk slowly, but also they listen attentively to a foreign doctor's broken English. One morning I surprise Dr. Dominges, the attending physician, because when he greets me with "Good morning," I reply, "Good morning, Dr. Dominges, I'm so far so good." But I cannot say phrases like "Thank you" and "You're welcome" for a long time. We don't use such expressions in Korea, and a custom developed over a lifetime is hard to change. I feel as if I am becoming anti-Korean.

One day, after almost two months have passed, I go into the bathroom in the hospital. I always wear my Seiko wristwatch, which is a necessity. I wash my hands, taking the watch off and putting in on the bathroom sink, and then I forget to put it back on. But I realize in a few minutes that I have left it behind. When I run back, it is nowhere to be found. I think I will certainly find it because in Korea, America is known as a paradise without any thieves or criminals. But here I experience my first pilferer in America.

Here, Hyun A, I notice that the men are tall, big, and in general, have very hairy bodies. The women are manly. They walk like men, lively and strong; they talk and laugh as loudly as men do; they smoke and drink like men. They wear pants—long or short—and like men they put their hands in their pockets while they are conversing or smoking. When they are hot, they all—men and women—take their shirts off; men show their bare chests; women their arms and armpits and deep down their front chests. In contrast to Korea, here there exists no virtue in shyness, modesty, and silence. American virtue seems to be the reverse: do whatever one pleases. Americans are free of inhibitions. They seem as free as birds in the sky.

When I rotate in the Emergency Room, the head of the department is from India and stresses that this is an emergency room for emergency care. For that reason he insists that we take a patient's history very briefly and promptly give proper care to him. Follow-up care and instructions should be left to his own attending physician. I am required to interpret an electrocardiogram and x-ray films instantly, especially during the night. Regardless of the night or day, patients constantly flow in and out of the emergency room. On duty late one night, the ER personnel order pizzas to enjoy during their break. Miss Klimchuk hands me a piece, saying, "This is called a pizza, a very popular fast food; everything—cheese, peppers, meat, onions, mushrooms—are on it. You just eat it, holding it like this. You don't need a fork." I smile and hold it. It smells like herbs, more like herb medicine than food. One piece is enough for me. Incessant radio music fills the ER. It is the FM stereo, reporting the weathercast and playing classical music. That radio keeps stirring my sense of sadness and solitude.

As the days roll by, my puny prestige and proud ego are injured because no one recognizes that I was a specialist in obstetrics and gynecology, as well as a teacher in Kwangju Girls High School, an instructor in Chosun University Women's College, and an instructor at the Nursing School of Chonman Medical School. Nobody here treats me with respect as an elder person and celebrity as in Korea. Here everyone treats me as nothing more than one of the interns. For a while, I am increasingly aggrieved by that treatment. But I shudder and wake up from my nightmare of misjudgment. I tell myself, "Who cares that you were the queen in Korea? You are here officially hired as an intern in this hospital. If you don't want to be treated as an intern, why are you here? You wanted to be here as an intern, St. Vincent Hospital didn't especially want you. Then what's wrong that they should treat you like any other intern?" Thus, my right judgment blows away and heals my injured swollen ego. No more grumbling!

However, unlike the other interns, my motherly instinct calls for my cubs. My flowing tears soak the pillow. In a letter that came a few days ago, your grandmother wrote to me that Steve has been ill from lung disease. His pediatrician took x-rays and gave him pills. He was stable, but he refused to take the cooked duck which was recommended by his doctor, saying it was too greasy. My baby, Robert, is now running around, not toddling any more. Luckily he doesn't miss us much, which makes your grandmother happy. You are doing exceptionally well at both school and home, helping your grandmother and two brothers as much as you can. I am an unnatural daughter to your grandmother: I put my heavy burden upon her shoulders in her old age. It tortures me too.

Not too long ago, by accident, I found a small picture by Kauss in which an older, barefooted sister piggybacks her little baby sister and stands on a ridge of a hill. The parents are farming on that hill. The hot summer breeze flings back the girl's black skirt and apron and long hair. I bought the picture at a small supermarket and hung it on my bedroom wall to remind me of you. I imagine you are piggy-backing your little brother Robert like the girl in the picture. When I see the two, I feel better. No matter how much distance separates a mother from her children, human motherly instinct knows no distance between them.

In November, your daddy joins me by transferring from the University of North Dakota to the University of Toledo, Ohio. He enrolls as a postgraduate to take a master's degree in political science. His coming lessens my tears at night as well as strengthens my brain and limbs in the day.

After I finish my rotation in the Department of Hematology, Dr. Richard Schafer, the head of the department, says, "You have done your job well, overcoming the language difficulties. But foreign doctors see only the luxurious aspects of America. Contrary to the general concept of foreigners, not all Americans are rich; many millions are short of food and clothing; many millions are homeless. I'll show you today the poverty in America." He takes me to the Uncle Sam Restaurant on Cherry Street, close to St. Vincent Hospital. In front of the restaurant there is a tall statue of Uncle Sam. Dr. Schafer treats me to a hamburger and French fries and ice cream.

Then he drives through the area. In the yards around the houses, the grass grows wantonly; windows are broken; the paint on the houses peels away; litter is scattered everywhere; some people sit drinking on the steps of their houses; liquor bottles and beer bottles are thrown on the porches and by the sidewalks. None of the houses are kept neatly. The people in the streets seem languid, indifferent, and joyless. He drives out of the area and brings me back to the hospital. "That's it. Keep up your good work. Good-bye," says he, and he drives out of the hospital. He is a great preceptor, teaching interns and residents what they are supposed to learn, taking them with him on his rounds. He lets us review the slides of interesting cases and read the referral articles. And now I know he is a great human soul, too.

Around the end of the internship, I take the Basic Medical Science examination that is held at the University of Michigan. This is not mandatory but tests how well I know basic medical science. I pass that examination.

Thus my one-year internship is brought to an end on June 25, 1970. The ceremony takes place at the hospital auditorium. I receive a letter of commendation as an outstanding intern from Edward F. Ockuly, MD, the Chief of Staff. In the envelope there is $25.00 in addition to the letter. It is priceless; I wouldn't trade it for millions. My one year of internship in the USA is the most arduous battlefield on which I have ever fought.

I have earned a one-week vacation. I am for the first time completely free from duty. On that afternoon, your daddy and I go downtown on foot since we don't have a car. We enter a White Castle restaurant and we eat a hamburger This is the most delicious hamburger I have ever tasted. That night I read my first novel in America, *The Goldenrod.* I tell your daddy that after the year of my struggle, I have gained the confidence to win the battle in the medical field in America. So we can bring our children to America, and we will give them glorious opportunities for their future. Your daddy agrees with me, brimming with joy. Thus, our first year in America ends well, and we decisively cross the Rubicon River to face a long American life.

§   §   §

Now the fresh new world is waiting for me. I see behind me the mountain that I have just surmounted; yet ahead of me lie other, higher peaks. I become a first-year OB & Gyn. resident in St. Vincent's Hospital. Everything is familiar to me: the systems of the hospital, the attending physicians, my fellow residents, the hospital personnel, even the food in the cafeteria. The knowledge and skill I gained during my residency in Korea soothe my nerves and muscles as I begin. However there are enormous fundamental dissimilarities in the practice of medicine here as contrasted with Korea. There is a wide variety of new knowledge, techniques, and treatments to explore. Best of all, America has the most advanced medical knowledge, techniques, tools, and authorities in all the world. More blessings are in the USA because here there are ample materials and new medicines to put into practice new ideas.

The basic difference between the United States and Korea in the system of medical practice is this: if any physician in Korea wants to open a medical practice, he must have his own hospital with beds for in-patients like a miniature of an American hospital. When he sees patients who are beyond his capabilities, he refers them either to a medical school hospital or to other specialized private doctors. Every patient has to pay with his own cash. There is no medical insurance in Korea. Therefore, people cannot afford to be ill. If they are sick, they try first to treat their symptoms themselves and wait and see, unless they are in a life-threatening situation.

I am getting comfortable in using the forceps dexterously in cases of difficult deliveries. My knowledge and skills to give anesthesia—both spinal and general anesthesia—have been expanded after two months' rotation in the Department of Anesthesia. Once, while on anesthesia rotation in the operating room, I am giving general anesthesia to a patient for an abdominal hysterectomy, holding the big black rubber bag and rhythmically squeezing it. To chase the reek of my garlic breath away, I put a stick of chewing gum in my mouth; I chew it intermittently. The chief of the Department of OB & Gyn. sees me; he instantly shoots a contemptuous glance at me, seemingly saying, "You are already Americanized! And in a bad way!" That needle is still in my brain, and it is hard to pluck it out.

Once the day that you and your two brothers are coming to us is set, nothing is the same. My heart and feet are in the air like floating balloons that hardly touch the ground. Your daddy's Lebanese friend, a postgraduate in the same political science department, drives us to the Toledo Airport on the day you arrive, August 14, 1971. It is a sultry afternoon.

When I see the white airplane rolling slowly in toward the terminal and stopping, all of a sudden a children's fable makes sense. A little son asks his mother who brought his newborn baby sister to his house; his mother tells him that a stork brought did. That's right! That's not just a tale but that is happening here, now. The giant white bird, the steel stork with two steel wings, brings our three children to us from Korea to America. The bird has crossed the Pacific Ocean and a thousand mountains and plains. What a long, long journey!

On the portable staircase, people are stepping down to the ground. You come to the top of the staircase. As your purple dress and your brothers' white tops and navy short pants and white sailor caps come into view, my heart begins to flutter in my chest. It is difficult to calm it down until you come down and we hug you. It seems we have been apart more than ten years rather than only fourteen months. You bring your two brothers all by yourself—you are only thirteen, Steve is six, Robert is three. As soon as I see the three of you, I go to Robert to hug him. Do you know what happens? He is crying and rushes back to you because he does not know who I am. This breaks my heart and causes me to burst into tears.

When your daddy joined me in Toledo, he rented a one-bedroom apartment across the street from St. Vincent Hospital for my convenience while we waited for postgraduate housing. In the meantime, he rides his bicycle or the city bus to the University of Toledo for school. The apartment is an old red-brick three-story building, covered with soot as if it was at one time in a fire. Its wooden gray staircase is attached to the side of the building. We receive you in that tiny apartment. There, in that small room and kitchen, having all our family together, we rebuild our home in America.

We have suddenly separated you from your grandma and your friends and put all of you in an utterly strange land, people, language, and environment. Your daddy and I have predicted that initially you will have a difficult time, as did we. Yet unexpected things happen. You are grown up and know the difference in countries; a queer situation is easier for Steve than for his little brother. But Robert still does not understand who I am; therefore, he calls and calls only for your grandma, especially during the night, crying, "Take me to grandma, take me to grandma...." He confuses day and night—it is day here but in Korea it is night. He stubbornly begs me to take him to his grandma. He can't understand because he is so little. I have to rest and sleep for the next day of work. One night or two I can tolerate, but I can no longer function without sleep. So, Hyun A, do you know what I do? On the fourth night, I bring home a liquid barbiturate; I give him a few drops and he sleeps, and I finally get a night's rest. Imagine what happens to him after one week in America! Robert needs the barbiturate no more than two nights; he stops crying and calling for his grandma. He sleeps at night; he plays during the day. Best of all, he acknowledges me as his mother. After he calls me "Mom" he completely forgets his grandma. What a blessing of simple minds children have!

Now my work is becoming my interest rather than my burden. I am immersed in choosing among diversified surgical techniques, perfecting bedside manners, or approaching the right treatments from many different attending doctors. No two doctors are alike. One morning Dr. Levin has a scheduled repeat C-section. He lets me do the appendectomy all by myself after he has finished the Caesarean delivery. Knowing how he does an appendectomy, I follow his way. This new experience elates me. I follow up the patient closely with him; she is dismissed in good condition without any complications.

We have some opportunity to socialize with the doctors. The OB & Gyn *Residents' Journal* meeting is held at Dr. Frederick Bawdle's. It is an evening so bitterly cold that both air and ground are frozen, but the bare trees stand still since the wind is quiet. The doctor's living room is snugly warm and brightened with a few lamps. On the white walls are large pictures of English royal fox hunting, a scene of the vast lake with a flight of wild geese, and family portraits. A Christmas wreath with dried vine tendrils and a large red ribbon is hung on the corner wall. The thick beige carpet and beige couches and love seat hedge the white-legged glass coffee table. The room reflects Dr. Bawdle's tidy and calm and gentle personality. At the end of the meeting, Mrs. Bawdle brings us freshly brewed coffee and freshly baked apple pie that is still hot. This is the best apple pie I have tasted in America.

Hyun A, children's fates—while they are totally dependent on their parents—are subject to their parents' destiny. You and your two brothers must blaze your way in the entirely alien soil of America. Shortly after you arrive, we move into the graduates' housing project on the campus of the University of Toledo at Secor and Bancroft Streets. The total number of students at the University is approximately 12,000, and the graduates' housing projects holds one hundred married families. Each house has two units, each with separate entrances and two bedrooms. Half of them are occupied by American graduates, the other by foreign graduates. They come from Korea, China, India, Pakistan, Lebanon, Europe, and South America, but predominantly from India. There are only two Korean families, but we are close neighbors—only two houses apart. These houses huddle together on the hill by the tower of the Administration Building. In between the curving road and the front houses is a green lawn with scattered young maple and mountain ash trees. Our unit is on the hilltop and commands a fine view of the campus.

Hyun A, our priority now is to send you and Steve to school. Your daddy finds that Old Orchard is our district school. You enter the seventh grade, Steve the first grade. In this period—nay, in most of his life with children in America—your daddy plays two roles: father and mother, for I am tied up with my duties at the hospital, leaving home early and coming home late. Furthermore, he has to be a good student to attain his master's degree in Political Science. Hyun A, believe me, he does everything to help all of you to grow well. He does his best without useless grumbles or slippery excuses.

During the first several weeks, when you return from school, you are frustrated and crying. One day one of the three daughters of Mr. Ma, a Chinese graduate student, runs to our house shouting that Steve has been tied to a tree by naughty neighbor boys. Your daddy flings open the door and rushes to the tree near our house. Four or five boys run away, but your daddy knows who two of the boys are: one is the son of a law student, the other the son of a chemistry student. Your daddy sees our Steve is crying, and he unties him and carries him home in his arms. Your daddy waits until after 6:00 p.m. because the two boys' fathers will be home by that time. He visits them and informs them that their sons did an unforgivable mischief to our Steve. Both fathers are greatly surprised to hear of such doings. They deeply apologize—bowing deeply—for their sons' bad behavior. Your daddy accepts the apology. After that Steve and the boys become good friends, playing together happily.

It never rains but it pours. Hyun A, when I am back home, your daddy tells me about Steve's first day of school. When he took Steve and put him in his classroom and was about to leave, Steve became very upset and wanted to leave with your daddy. He could not understand why your daddy could not sit with him in the class. He cried, but your daddy explained that he must stay in the class with his teacher and his classmates. Probably to Steve everyone in the class was strange-looking and different from his friends in Korea; he was unable to understand what the students were saying; he could not speak to them in English. So your daddy waited outside the classroom. But he never came out during the class hour, and your daddy brought him home. On the second day of school, Steve doesn't resist entering the classroom.

There is another hurdle for Steve. At the end of the week, before your daddy, he cries and cries after coming home from school. Your daddy asks, "Why are you crying?"

"I am not on the baseball team. Other boys play, but I cannot play," he answers. Crying is a very powerful language, especially when no speech can communicate. The next day, your daddy visits Steve's teacher. He tells her of Steve's situation.

"Steve came late from Korea. Our baseball team was already organized before his coming," she says. So your daddy visits the principal's office and meets the principal, Mr. Henderson, and explains that Steve is unhappy because he can't play baseball—the teacher has already organized the team. If the teacher puts Steve on the team, she would displace one of the members from the team. After listening to the story, the principal calls the teacher to his room and says, "Mrs. Joseph, don't stick to a nine-member team, add one more. Steve just came from Korea; he wants to play with the other boys. "All right, I'll try," she answers, and she puts Steve on the baseball team immediately. From then on he plays baseball or any other sport that the other boys play. He is recognized as an excellent athlete by his principal, his teacher, and his friends.

Hyun A, your daddy and I are not always available; you don't have any friend to talk to. At school, you don't understand what your teacher is saying or what your classmates are saying. You are unable to read and do the homework; you feel helpless, like a bird with clipped wings. In part your bitter cry is that in Korea you always had a leading role in your class as a class monitor or president, but here, suddenly, you are a nobody. It's a good thing that you never give in to just sitting and crying. You not only study until late at night but you find the way to solve your problems.

After school, you go to Mrs. Yang's, the only Korean family on the campus, and you help her with her two children, a girl of five and a boy of two. Both Mr. and Mrs. Yang are highly educated and of a noble Korean family. Mr. Yang is here to study for a Ph.D. in chemistry; Mrs. Yang is a housewife who graduated from the Yee Hwa Women's College in Seoul. She is able to speak and to read English fluently. Now she is raising her children and keeping house. She and you get along well, and she becomes your tutor. When she goes out, you baby-sit for her children. She and Mr. Yang teach you English and American customs. Both are extraordinarily kind and considerate people. Through your determined struggle and our steady encouragement, your frustration and crying diminish by degrees.

After two months you make new friends; you understand better what your teacher says and what the books say. In the meantime, your teacher, Mrs. Howard, supports you a great deal: when you draw pictures in art class, she hangs your pictures—of course your drawings deserve to be hung. Moreover, your talent in solving mathematical problems promotes your morale, since figures, signs, and symbols are universal. Another wonderful asset is your athletic ability. Since you were a little girl you have been good at all kinds of sports. When you were in the sixth grade at Syusuck Elementary School—the second biggest elementary school in Korea, with three thousand students—you were the master of ceremonies at the regular gymnastic hour, standing in front of a microphone on the high podium. Thus whenever you have ball games or races, you have no problems; your keen eyes and quick hands and running legs speak for you. By the end of the first semester, you are more and more interested in school.

Besides your and Steve's schooling, your daddy sends Robert to preschool to familiarize him with the new language and strange environment. Because of this, Robert doesn't have the problems that you and Steve had to go through. Robert plays, sings, and draws well with his friends both at school and at home.

In the middle of May 1971, your grandmother joins us in America. After the three of you came to America, I wrote to her that we were having difficult times: Steve was tied up to the tree by the neighbor boys, and you were crying, and Robert had to be put in daycare because your daddy and mom had to work. She instantly answered that although the process to get a passport to come to America would take a long time, she could not be happy while her children were suffering. For that reason, she would like to come and stay with us and help us until your daddy should complete his Ph.D. Your grandmother knew—both by what she had heard and had seen in Korean of foreign families—that she could expect a miserable time here in the United States within the invisible fence formed by language and custom, having nobody to speak to and nowhere to go.

My brother and sisters and uncles and aunts all objected to her going to America. But your grandmother was determined to come to America to help us, ignoring her own comfort. Who will sacrifice their easy and comfortable life in old age for their children? They would be our parents from whom we inherited our blood. Especially, it is your grandmother, whose priority in her lifetime has been her children. We cannot help feeling fortunate to have inherited your grandmother's great spirit. Her presence in our home brightens our dark period and restores order and peace in our disorganized and stressful house, giving everyone a sense of being loved and secure in her or his work and position: your daddy can concentrate on his studies, I can concentrate on my work, and you and your brothers feel home is a place to talk and to laugh and to eat as much as you like. Anyway, you all have been inseparably attached to your grandmother since you were little. Your grandmother's joining us gives us a peaceful and happy home in America.

One morning after the first year of your schooling here is over, your daddy brings us the *Toledo Blade* and proudly shows us a feature article about your amazing achievement. Your story and your photograph occupy one whole page in the "Living" section of the newspaper. In the second semester of school you have straight A's in all your subjects—this from knowing nothing about English, not even the English alphabet—one year ago. Your teacher and principal were so impressed by your achievement that the principal called a news writer at the *Toledo Blade* and had him interview you in his office. Now you are the pride of the school. You become our pride too. Great teachers give every opportunity to their students; good students achieve their goals by struggling hard and making the most of their opportunities.

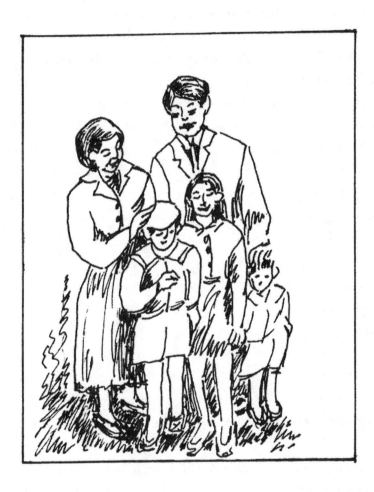

Thus we complete our first year in our new land successfully and happily.

—14—

New Medical Training, New Customs

Dear Hyun A,

Now your daddy acquires his Master's degree from the Political Science Department at Toledo University. He desires to continue his study for the doctorate; however, UT doesn't offer his program. He is accepted in the Ph.D. program at Wayne State University in Detroit, Michigan, and I by St. John's Hospital, also in Detroit. Again, our family must face a new place to live and new people to meet. We expect to endure extra effort and stress until adjustments are made. Nonetheless, this time we all feel much less burdened since all our family is together to share some of the hin-

drance as well as to become more accustomed to the English language and American customs.

 We move into a low-rent apartment located close to St. John's
Hospital. All three of you children are sent to the district school. St.
John's Hospital is a Catholic hospital, one of the biggest in east Detroit. It is located on Morris Road at Seven Mile Road in the vicinity
of Grosse Pointe, an exclusive area that overlooks Lake Erie and where
wealthy people live. The hospital has more than eight hundred beds
for the admission patients. Its Department of Pathology is well known
nationwide. For this reason, Dr. James S. Humes, the Chairman, was
selected to do the autopsy of John F. Kennedy after his assassination.
The hospital chapel attached to the rear of the hospital is as large and
as beautifully ornamented as a regular church. In the Department of
OB & Gyn there are about sixty attending physicians who deliver
three thousand babies annually. The hospital has a four-year residency
program; two residents in each year bring a total of eight residents
to the OB & Gyn. Department. I am brought in as one of the two
second-year residents. My partner, Dr. Hanna, is a male doctor who
was a practicing surgeon in Egypt before coming to this hospital. The
one female resident besides me, Manuela Ocompo, is a first-year
resident.

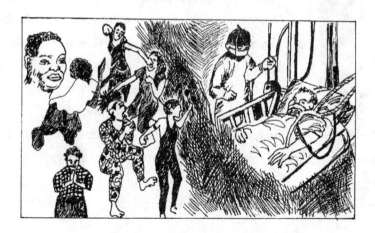

In order to deliver these thousands of babies, the obstetric section in the hospital occupies considerable space: two wings of the hospital on the second floor, the east wing for deliveries and C-sections, the south for the labor rooms. The east wing of the first floor is for the Outpatient Clinic OB & Gyn. patients. Early every Saturday morning before starting work, there is always a residency meeting for journal review as well as presentation of cases and discussion. All the departments of the hospital are so active and lively. During weekdays—even on Saturday mornings, early morning or at lunch hour—the hospital auditorium is occupied for some type of academic conferences: radiology, internal medicine, pediatric, surgery, and lab. Gynecologic surgery cases in the operating rooms continue every day. The whole personality of the hospital created by all the physicians and workers seems pulsing towards the patients pouring in, striving to give them the best, the most effective care.

The atmosphere of the hospital and my own OB & Gyn. department's constant flux of patients with newborn babies, plenty of gynecologic surgical cases requiring diverse techniques, and the need for different approaches to face their patients and problems by the gynecologic surgeons animate my interest in my job. The surgeons seem to be happy and humorous. They talk and laugh all the time whenever they get together. One day in the operating room, I am scrubbing for Dr. Welson's vaginal hysterectomy case. As he holds up his forearms to drain the Lysol water and to pass me to enter the OR, he says close to my ear, "Don't you like me?" For I keep silent and do my work.

Hyun A, Dr. Panfilo DiLoreto, the head of the Department of OB & Gyn., is of Italian descent, a gray-haired father figure in his mid sixties, rather short, with hearty and hale build and large eyes and large hands. Under him all the residents learn to be frugal surgeons. Whenever we scrub in his surgery case, we cannot use any catgut suture thread more than two inches long—for the maximum utilization of these threads—and we cannot leave these fragments of threads on the operating field. We cannot leave the gauze that wiped up blood in the operation area. "Make your mess in your own house, not here!" he stings us. "Pick up that suture, use it again!" He truly applies his simple, humble, appreciative philosophy to his own life: when he dines, he never leaves any food on his plate—not even one grain of rice. However, on special occasions he invites all the residents, even their little children, to his house, offering food in a setting of glittering sterling silver and fine china.

As my busy months pass by, my fingers no longer tremble when I give my clinic patients spinal anesthesia. Under the attending preceptors, we residents see and treat—either medically, surgically, or obstetrically—and follow up our own clinic patients. Also the preceptors let us become involved in the surgery and care of their own patients and do not use us merely to hold retractors and wipe up blood. The more involved in the patient care, the more interested we residents become. Thus, I am wrapped in a whirl of one bustling year with enthusiasm and bright prospects.

During the summer, before three months of rotation to our pathological department, I have to go downtown to the Receiving General Hospital in Detroit, forty-five miles to the west. In this part of the city poverty-stricken black people are crowded together. Because of demographic distribution, socio-economic conditions, and many drug-addicts in the population, here there are terrible diseases that we do not often see at St. John's: for example, the pelvic inflammatory disease, ectopic pregnancy, sexually transmitted diseases, actual or alleged rape cases, or psychiatric illness.

On my first day's duty at the Emergency Room, I am shocked to see the sight of real living pandemonium: under a searing sun, on the semicircular driveway to the ER entrance, several carts are lined up waiting for their turn. Patients are tied to the steel rail of the cart with white cloths, moaning and groaning and twisting. One of them, a middle-aged man in great distress, wriggles and shouts to be free. A young woman with disheveled hair and unbuttoned blouse sits on the white sheet covering her cart, fumbling with a dirty towel and muttering and babbling to herself endlessly. The ambulance siren is screaming and rushing to the ER entrance; the ambulance staff are carrying a bloody stretcher, squeezing an airbag for a gunshot wound patient.

The ER is divided into many sections of treatment rooms by beige draperies; on the white walls is life-saving equipment—oxygen supply, respirators. All the rooms are being used: cardiac conversion, resuscitation, suturing, EKG, gastric irrigation, pelvic examination. The whole ER bursts at the seams with sick patients and their families, doctors, nurses, nurses' aids, and policemen: it resounds with the discordant sounds of crying and groaning and running footsteps and the urgent voices of the patients, the doctors, the nurses.

On a typical night call, four to seven alleged rape cases show up at the ER. With each case I have to examine the patient using the rape kit, collecting evidence by pelvic and physical examination, which requires a lot of time and sometimes consumes the entire night. One time I suture the deeply lacerated vaginal wall of a seventy-five-year-old victim who has been robbed and raped by a young robber. Another time a young mother brings in her five-year-old daughter, claiming the child has been raped by the daughter's stepfather. The little girl holds her teddy bear in her arms and is sucking a lollipop. Very often we perform surgeries in relation to ectopic pregnancy and PID and fibroid uterus. Sexually transmitted diseases and rape victims are by far the most frequent cases seen here. In contrast, at St. John's Hospital we see only a few ectopic pregnancies in a year; PID is seen less often; the alleged rape cases are rare. Instead, at St. John's, we see diabetes, gallstones, breast and uterine and ovarian cancer, or endometriosis. This short training period is invaluable to me in showing me another aspect of the medical world in America.

§   §   §

Now, you and your brothers are growing. You have to go to high school, and you all need more space to play and study in your own house with your own yard. Your daddy buys a house for our family at Harperwood, which is a ten-minute drive to St. John's Hospital. You enroll in Harperwood School; so do your brothers.

The Harperwood area is highly populated. Houses with three bedrooms and two-car garages of regular size are side by side without much space in between. Strings of them are on every street like beads on a rosary. The streets are clean, and an array of trees cast their cool shadows upon the sidewalk; every house's lawn is green and well kept; summer flowers surround the house and flowers in vibrant pots hang at the porch. Our house is on Woodmont Street, several houses away from the main freeway. It is naturally bright and warm since it faces south and is exposed to the sun all day long.

Right behind our back yard is Harperwood Memorial Park, surrounded by green grass. People here enjoy the park, playing with slides, monkey bars, seesaws, a rocking horse, and a jogging trail. At the center of the park is a round pond. In the winter, its water freezes and offers the best possible ice rink, naturally made. It has a magnetic beauty and power to draw the district children even in the depth of the freezing winter. They are wrapped up with snow or ski gear and knitted caps and mittens. The little ones hold their mothers' or fathers' hands. Their multicolored attire—black, red, green, yellow, and blue—adds to the lively moving. Sometimes heavy falling snow whitens them all.

When winter comes, this pond is made for Robert. Of course, you and Steve are good skaters, but not as good as Robert. When he puts on his black ski gear and his red Santa cap and long red scarf and red mittens and gets into the ring, he pushes himself to slide forward smoothly and swiftly, swings around, and races through the crowds of children. When he does so, the white wool ball at the tip of his cap swings like a pendulum; his long frilled scarf flies around his neck. A little cardinal seems flying in the snow-falling sky. I think—maybe this statement is parental prejudice—he is the best among all the children playing, and he skates like a professional. His style, beauty, and agile movement as a little child are all but perfect. Just watching Robert play gives us immense pleasure. The unending sounds of ice cracking, as well as children's jolly screams, fill the gray air of winter in Harperwood.

Conveniently, the back edge of this Harperwood Memorial Park borders on the parking lot of the Hudson Shopping Mall, which includes JC Penny and other stores. We can walk for shopping; the three of you walk to school. One summer Saturday afternoon, when I come back from the hospital, the three of you are cleaning the garage and arranging a table and chairs and glass pitchers. You sweep our concrete driveway and porch. "What's going on here?" I ask.

"My teacher said we have to help the disadvantaged and the sick," Steve says. "Cancer Foundation Day is tomorrow. We want to make money by selling lemonade at our garage tomorrow." On Sunday midmorning the announcement on the card—Please stop by for cool lemonade! 50C per cup!—is already up in our front yard by the sidewalk. The table is covered with a red-and-white-checked table cloth, lemonade pitchers and bottles and paper cups and paper napkins. After church, the children on the street are gathering; knowing the kids' purpose, some adults stop and buy lemonade. Amazing! At the end of the day, you have earned $23.00. The next day Steve hands over the total amount to his teacher; we guess he pleases his teacher. Best of all, he and Robert and you for the first time experience a great lesson in how to help the disadvantaged and the sick.

Hyun A, you have an Easter vacation when you are a junior at Harperwood High School. You ask your daddy and mom to buy a paint box and brushes for drawing pictures, and your daddy buys what you need. Much to our surprise, we discover you have a natural endowment through your multitude of drawings: Picasso's pictures of still life, seascapes, landscapes, and portraits. I bring your portfolio to St. John's Hospital to show Dr. C. Lee, who is our chief resident in OB & GYN as well as a poet and a connoisseur. He praises your talent and recommends that you pursue a career in art, applying at a special art school after you graduate from high school. While he is appreciating your work, two attending physicians pass by; they admire your skill and talent. Dr. Lee wants of have one of your pictures, a copy of Picasso's musicians, to hang in his living room. The other two doctors also ask for pictures. I let them have what they want. Later on Dr. Lee and Dr. Hummel invite all the residents in OB & GYN to their homes; I see your pictures hung in the center of their living rooms, which makes me proud. When I tell you about this event, you feel highly flattered. It is natural that you feel that way, for every artist loves to have such positive feedback.

Despite Dr. Lee's advice that you should go to art school, your daddy doesn't want you to; to become a renowned artist requires an immense amount of time and energy. You would have a terribly difficult time; you would not make a living unless you became a remarkable artist. Your daddy wants you to have a secure profession. If you want to pursue a career as an artist, probably years later, when your children are grown up, you might try. You agree with your daddy and decide to go the University of Michigan after you finish high school.

(Hyun A, I have never told you about this: while you are in medical school, your daddy and I visit your uncle in Chicago in late summer. After dinner all four of us—daddy uncle, aunt, myself—sit in the living room and turn our conversation to family affairs and family members. From across the room I see a small framed picture hung on the wall right beside the front door. It is a magnificent piece, radiating the tranquillity of a gleaming, dusky ocean that stretches to the twilit horizon; on the beach is the dark silhouette of a woman against the sky's afterglow. "Sister Myogyung, that picture is so beautiful there! Where did you buy it?" I ask. She smiles and says, "You did not know? Really? It was Hyun A's. A few years back, your brother asked her for it. Most of our guests notice it and praise the artist's uncommon talent." Not only do your uncle and aunt acknowledge that you have artistic aptitude but reaffirm what your daddy and mom already know.)

At the beginning of that same summer vacation, you ask your daddy to buy you a sewing machine, for you want to sew for yourself and your grandmother. Your daddy initially doubts if you will use the machine, but you please with your initiative to try something new. He buys you a brand new Singer sewing machine with two brown wrought-iron legs and a wide pedal. You easily follow the patterns, cut the fabric, and not only tailor your own clothes but your grandmother's. Helping with her chores, learning cookery—your grandmother is a gourmet cook, as you know—talking with her freely in Korean while your two brothers are unable to speak the Korean language well, you are always your grandmother's best friend.

Moreover, after you start sewing, you give pleasure and a spurt of your energy to your grandma. She spends her time in a much more lively way, designing her own patterns with a variety of colorful pieces of fabric for making quilts for your brothers. (She made one for you, too, but in the second year of college at your dormitory, somebody stole it from your room. You must have cried when that theft happened, thinking back to how hard your grandma worked for you.) When you leave home, your daddy is her best friend, taking time to listen to her, to talk to her, to ask her what she wants and needs. She does not have anyone to speak to except us. Your daddy knows she has been sacrificing herself for all of us. Because of her, without worrying about the three of you at home, your daddy has been able to concentrate on his studies; he obtains the best scholarship available for the Ph.D. program students. This is a happy time for us: all our family on the weekends go to the park and picnic or visit the Detroit zoo; on Sundays we go to the Presbyterian Church; on our way home, your daddy takes us to a restaurant for lunch. Going to church, the park, the zoo on weekends becomes the center of our family life.

One Sunday after the church service is over, we are invited to dinner by an Italian family, the Pizzenos. A stunningly good-looking man, Mr. Pizzeno is married to a Korean woman; they have one seven-year-old son. All six of us, and Mr. Pizzeno's father, are the dinner guests. Mrs. Pizzeno sets up the dining table with a clean tablecloth, napkins, tablemats, and silverware. To our surprise she cooks gourmet Italian foods better than a real Italian: spaghetti sauce with meatballs, spaghetti, genuine sesame seed Italian bread, baked cheese potato casserole, a creamy mushroom-string-bean casserole, and authentic Italian cookies and Canoli and ice cream for dessert. We all eat our fill of this scrumptious Italian meal

Then right after dinner at the table, the father asks Mr. Pizzeno for a cigarette. The son takes a cigarette out of his cigarette pack and throws it on the table towards his father. The father picks it up and smokes without any words of reproach for his son's behavior or any change of color in his face. I am amazed to see the son's behavior towards his father! In Korea, if a father wants to smoke, a son politely stands up, walks to him, gives him a cigarette, and lights it for him courteously. According to our long Korean tradition, children are not permitted to smoke in front of their parents. However, Mr. Pizzeno is very kind and friendly and considerate to his father, wife, son, and other people. I realize that this is a cultural, customary difference in a different country rather than rude behavior. Many of the customs in America are different from what I'm used to.

§   §   §

During my residency, I often have to work at night. During night call, the night-duty nurses and I work together, sharing all kinds of ideas, friendship, food, activities, gossip, and customs. The night itself makes us feel close, like family. Outside the hospital the world is dark and silent except for droning cars running on the Moross Road. Inside the hospital after midnight the OB floor is dimmed and silent. We look like crows on the oak's branch; they are few, but always together. We women talk. Mrs. McKimm says, "Although we women dress up like queens, if we do not wear jewels. we seem to miss a great part of finery. We ladies have the right to be beautiful and to wear fine jewels. I love to show mine; I think they make me feminine and are something to cherish and treasure."

"That is true," says Mrs. Peltcher. "My ears were pierced when I was five. My Aunt Nancy did it for me; she gave me gold ball earrings. Dr. Yoo, you must have your ears pierced. If you feel uncomfortable wearing earrings all the time, you can just put them on when you really need them."

One night, Mrs. Keck brings her tools for piercing ears. She is an artist. Not only has she an inborn gift but also she has infinite affection for her painting. From time to time she shares her art, bringing her thick portfolio in which landscapes, still lifes, and portraits are stacked. She has large, nostalgic, dreamy-blue eyes and a sharp nose on her freckled face. As she speaks, her whispering, husky voice becomes louder, causing the veins to engorge on her long ivory neck.

"Are you ready? Really ready?" says she. She draws her chair and gently pulls my left ear lobe close to the light. "Close your eyes!" With an alcohol sponge, she scrubs my earlobe—without any kind of agents to numb the skin—she swiftly drills through it bloodlessly and repeats the same procedure on the other earlobe. The result is that the right side hole is lower than the left side, but who will notice the one-and-a-half millimeter's difference?

When I saw Indians boring many holes through their body—especially at the nose, eyebrow, tongue, ears, and umbilicus—I thought they were savages to do such things. Now I feel that I have become one of them. But I have never regretted having done this. Life requires an extra adornment with sparkling stones and full feathers.

At the OB and Gyn. Clinic, under the supervision of the clinical instructors, we residents see and treat the patients or admit them and treat them medically or surgically. Our patients belong to the Medicaid governmental program that covers their medical problems, including prenatal care and delivery; they are supposed to be poor, without jobs or their own health insurance. St. John's Hospital accepts a large number of Medicaid patients, stretching out its benevolent hand to them. Ideally this system should be a good socio-medical program, but a considerable number of reckless and ignorant people abuse the welfare project. Many of them come to the clinic as often as they like; and despite giving them a regular appointment, they show up at any time of the day or night, either at the emergency room or at the clinic, without a good reason to see the doctors. For instance, a slight cold beginning with a runny nose, or a scratched knee, or a mild bruise from a fall will bring them to the hospital. They could take care of all of these problems by themselves at home.

If they had to pay their own medical expenses or if they were sensible, they would never allow themselves to come to the hospital. They should save those medical resources—which they are wasting—for other truly deserving patients. In one extreme case, I see a young, single woman who has had eight artificial abortions, all paid for by the government. Worst of all, she is utterly unaware of the peril to her health of having these abortions. She is remorseless and shameless, acting as if she is a privileged patient. The hospital and doctors are unable to stand up against such a patient's abusiveness. If they do, they would seem to oppose the patient's civil rights, and they would soon be buried by the overpowering flood of criticism and litigation.

Sometimes I see the patients who do have jobs and have medical insurance, but the insurance company doesn't cover medications and office visits as well as other minor procedures, and their income is too low for them to pay for what they need. So they have to suffer. They are the citizens who work day by day with their hands and feet, paying taxes, raising and educating their children with their own sweat. On the contrary, the Medicaid patients can come to see the doctors for anything at all, and can get any medication. I hope someday a better medical system will emerge.

When I become a senior resident, my accountability for both my duty as a chief resident and my own preparation for my future practice gets heavier and broader. First of all, the Department of Medical Education at St. John's Hospital has a distinctive program for an annual scientific seminar. This seminar has a twofold purpose: one is for the promotion of acquiring medical knowledge for all residents in the hospital; the other for the updated evaluation of the hospital patients' care and statistics. The reason is that every resident has to pick his material from the hospital patients' charts.

This year the title of my subject is "Intensive Care in High Risk Obstetrics." Since 1969, St. John's Hospital has set up the Department and Unit of Intensive Care in High Risk Obstetrics. Dr. Chang Lee is head of this department and has introduced fetal heart monitoring equipment, which allows obstetricians to diagnose fetal distress early and so save the babies. At this time, the use of the ultrasonogram along with the fetal monitoring cardiogram is a watershed event in obstetrical care. I collect materials on these new methods, and my evaluations show that using both ultrasonogram and fetal monitoring increases early detection of fetal distress, decreases the number of stillbirths, and results in higher Apgar scores in newborn babies. My study demonstrates that our High Risk OB Unit is worth having for the better care of our patients.

We residents select our different topics, and in our hospital auditorium we present our research papers including slides before all attending obstetricians. My presentation is chosen as the best one, and I am given the opportunity to present my material before all the hospital attending physicians and staff.

This spring I not only must prepare my presentation but I must also get a certification to practice medicine for myself in America. For that purpose, I must take the FLEX examination; anyone who passes this exam can practice in thirteen states without taking the individual state exam. I take the test and pass. And at the end of the fourth year of residency I take and pass the written board examination of Obstetrics & Gynecology. The final, hardest thing is how and where to find the place that I ought to settle and practice. I feel as if I am a wandering prospector in quest of gold.

Finally, on June 23, 1974, the day for the ceremony of the completed residency is held at the Yacht Club Ballroom at Grosse Pointe. Each resident's spouse or a friend is invited. Grosse Pointe is the community where the wealthy and privileged classes live. It commands a fine view of ever-blue Lake Erie with its yachts and sail-boats. On a regular day, ordinary people—not being Yacht Club members—are unable to get to the tennis courts or even to the restroom. Tonight, in the grand ballroom, several gigantic chande-liers on the high ceiling glitter like diamonds. Heavy royal-blue drap-eries are held open at the windows by thick gold tassels; the lacy curtains veil the window sills. The majestic paintings of English and French royal cotillions, the portraits of aristocratic gentlemen and ladies, and the bright scarlet carpet provoke a sense of grandiosity and splendor. The round dining tables are arranged with royal blue table cloths and napkins. The room bursts at the seams from the crowd.

At the end of the dining area is the head table, where many important people from the hospital face us. Dr. Rush holds the mi-crophone and extends a warm welcome to all attending guests and praises the great achievement of all the graduating residents. He pre-sides over the ceremony, handing out a certificate to each individual. Your daddy sits beside me and seems anxious, waiting for my turn. No sooner do I hear the sound of my name than my heart starts throbbing fast, and my feet falter as I step forward. Dr. Rush takes up a blue folder and reads my award to the audience:

St. John's Hospital Detroit Michigan
Annual Scientific Seminar Award
June 1974
Department Obstetrics & Gynecology
Chi Sun Yoo Rhee, M.D.

John M. O'Lane, M.D.   William E. Rush, M.D.
Department Chief   Director of Medical Education

He hands me the certificate and award with a white envelope. He smiles broadly and shakes my hand vigorously. "Congratulations on your great achievement!" he says. I receive a thunder of applause.

Hyun A, can you imagine how I feel at this moment, clutching the award in my hand and walking down that hall in front of all the guests? I wish I could show you that momentous event. For this one flashing moment no man in the whole world stands higher than I.

I must tell you one thing more. I wear the long dress that you tailored for me all by yourself just for this occasion. It is the classic style of a long evening dress. It is made of a soft, royal-purple fabric with large pink roses and has a low, round neckline, long sleeves, and a flaring skirt. As I reach our table, your daddy pulls out my chair for me. I open the envelope; you can never guess what's there! It is money; $50.00 for the award! It is an amount beyond measure!

Thus, my four years of residency are completed with rapture in my heart.

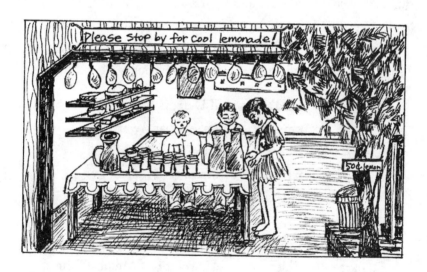

—15—

The Solo Medical Practice

Dear Hyun A,

The time has come. It is July, 1974. Being independent and standing alone as an obstetrician and gynecologist, I must now use the knowledge and skills I have perfected in the healing arts. It appears that my new beginning is like that of a pioneer who prepares for and has to defy a multitude of unknown difficulties; only his vision of a better world drives him to attempt his hurdles.

Among the many places to select from for my practice, predestination lands me in Monroe, Michigan. I have never even heard its name before. Why do I say "predestination?" It is my choice. Of all places, why do I come here to Monroe? If I had chosen any other place, my life would have turned out differently. From Grosse Pointe, Detroit, I drive south for ninety minutes and leave I-75 at the Monroe exit. From both sides of the highway as I approach the exit, patches of green woodlands spread like archipelagoes over the green fields that are merging into the far away horizon where farmhouses, barns, and granaries sprawl out sporadically. I take a road to North Monroe Street; even though it is a narrow, two-way road, it is one of the main roads of the city. The street is quiet except for an occasional passing car.

The small number of houses huddle together along the road and by the patches of woods on the farms. The gray, weather-worn, dilapidated barns stand forsaken on the fields near the road. The desolate environment with its sparse population dampens my bright enthusiasm. I feel like a défeated homecoming soldier. Further to the south, more houses come into sight, but there is not a single skyscraper, only a K-Mart at the crossroads. Eerily, amidst the houses, there is a cemetery right by he street; the small and large crowded gravestones stand fixed or lie flat within a tall black ironwork fence.

Further down to the south, the road is lined with houses, and North Monroe Street forms the thoroughfare with Elm Street. There is St. Mary's Catholic Church with a large, white statue of the Virgin Mary that is older than the date of American Independence. On the street opposite the church is a huge greenish brass statue of General Custer riding his horse. Both the church and the statue show the history and pride and spirit of Monroe City. Monroe Street extends to a concrete bridge crossing over the Raisin River and leads to the downtown area. The old store buildings of one or two or three stories stick together without any space in between, and there are no visible parking lots. However a few stately church towers above the city blocks spear into the sky. The scale of the downtown area is small. The city gives off the air of an old, quiet Catholic town. I know I can learn to love this place. I decide to practice here.

Before moving down to Monroe, your daddy and I must find a place to live. Hence, a realtor takes us to Hollywood Avenue because it is convenient to the hospital and my office; besides, the place is known for a good environment for families. When we walk up the street to see the house, two boys around ten or twelve years old ask, "Are you looking for a house to buy?"

"Yes," your daddy replies.

"No! We don't need you coming here!" the older boy shouts.

Even if those are a little child's words, after hearing this sentence, your daddy asks the realtor to find a house for us in another place. "When we lived on the east side of Detroit and Harperwood, all the residents were friendly and welcomed our coming to live with them. Why should we buy a house in a place hostile to foreigners? The children around Hollywood may treat our children with the same attitude," he says to the realtor. So Mr. Black finds a house on Ruff Drive where the neighbors are friendly and where our three children become friends with the neighbor's boys and girls immediately. Robert and Steve attend St. Michael's School in the second and fifth grades respectively; Hyun A the tenth grade at St. Mary's Academy.

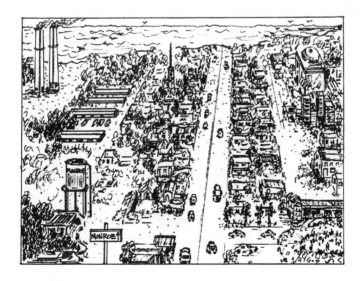

As time passes, I find the city is not what it seems. The more I learn about the city, the richer I find the features revealed behind its shabby veil. I find treasures hidden in unexpected places. The vast blue water of Lake Erie borders the east side of the city. The fertile farmlands encompass the city, supplying a cornucopia of crops, fruits and vegetables. On the far bank of the lake, the twin towers of the Fermi Nuclear Power Plant, like an alien planet, send white columns of smoke to the sky; on the bank opposite are two towering chimneys of the Detroit Edison Company. Their trails of dark gray smoke rise endlessly in the high spaces. Too, nationally known companies are here—the Consolidated Paper Company, the La-Z-Boy Chair Company, and the Monroe Auto Equipment Company. Furthermore, St. Mary's Academy and the convent are world-known educational institutions. Within an hour's drive from Monroe are the following schools: Wayne State University in Detroit, the University of Michigan in Ann Arbor, and the University of Toledo. The city's population is approximately 40,000-50,000, but in Monroe County it is 180,000.

Originally, in the city, two Catholic hospitals, Mercy and Memorial, provided for all the medical needs of the community. They were built half a mile apart; and in the past, general practitioners and family physicians cared for the ill, delivered babies, and performed surgeries in the two hospitals. Gradually more medical specialists have been required to care for local patients rather that referring them to nearby cities—Detroit, Ann Arbor, Toledo. In the late 1960's a surgeon, Dr. Ansari, built the multi-specialties' clinic called Monroe Clinic. Here new specialists in urology, ophthalmology, pediatrics, internal medicine, ear and nose and throat, obstetrics and gynecology have joined with Dr. Ansari. I am one of them.

Hyun A, I had a great advantage in being a woman in this small, conservative town. Many female patients prefer to visit female doctors. Moreover, two distinguished female general practitioners who had delivered thousands of babies in Monroe have just retired. It is a time when Monroe demands female physicians; I fill in their empty position and am welcomed warmly. Here, the total annual deliveries total about one thousand, which suggests a very busy OB department.

In the OB & Gyn. Department, three male obstetricians are using the labor and delivery rooms. Three male general practitioners also are involved in delivering babies; but shortly after my arrival, two of them quit delivering babies because of age and because of the increase in obstetric malpractice insurance premiums and increased litigation. However, one of the general practitioners wholeheartedly participates in delivering babies. Particularly, he seems to be an advocate of the new Lamaze method: prenatal classes, natural delivery, and the father acting as coach in the delivery room. He recommends that his mothers breast feed, primarily for the baby's health and secondarily for the bonding between mother and child.

Although within a hundred miles of the big city of Detroit, the ways of medical practice in the small city of Monroe are different from those of a big city. Here in Monroe, patients rarely request pain medication during their labor. They seem to blow away their torturous pain with a brown paper bag, using the technique learned in their Lamaze class. Unless there is a surgical delivery such as a C-section or a forceps delivery, physicians do not give spinal anesthesia. If it is needed, the physician has to give the spinal anesthesia by himself because the hospital has no anesthesiologist, only a group of nurse anesthetists who have given general anesthesia for surgery cases. Therefore, the person accountable for any bad side effects from the anesthesia is the physician, not the anesthetist. No obstetricians even attempt to apply the epidural anesthesia for controlling the pain of labor and delivery. I brought with me the special needle used for epidural anesthesia; I have never used it.

In the ward of the labor and delivery room, there is no isolated surgical room for the C-section. Therefore, whenever we have a C-section, the OB nurses notify the surgery crew in the operating room on the second floor; they bring a moving cart to the labor room on the third floor. It is very time-consuming and dangerous in an emergency situation for both a mother and a baby.

(In contrast, in St. John's Hospital, anesthesiologists gave spinal, epidural, and general anesthesia for the vaginal or abdominal deliveries. Most vaginal deliveries were performed under spinal anesthesia. For the pain of labor, a majority of patients were routinely given the pain medication by injection. The new Lamaze movement was not yet discussed here. As the Cesarean delivery room was set up next to the Labor and Delivery Room floor, the OB nurses scrubbed for the surgery and an anesthesiologist came up to give the anesthesia. This setup was far more convenient and faster. Finally, most mothers would prefer to give a bottle feeding rather than a breast feeding.)

Hyun A, in 1976 your daddy builds a new office building for me across North Macomb Street opposite Mercy Hospital. This is a great advantage for my practice, allowing me to have sufficient rooms and space and permitting patients to fill their prescriptions at the Professional Pharmacy, which is under our same roof. Since the hospital is right across the street, they can go there easily for their tests.

Shortly after moving into the new office, my office staff and I have an unexpected commotion. One late summer afternoon in the middle of office hours, a man rushes into the office through the waiting room, supporting his distressed wife. "My wife is in labor, her water has just broken, the baby is coming!" he gasps. All the patients stand up and rush to the agonized woman. The office instantly turns stormy. We all bring her—actually, all of us hold her—into the examination room and put her on the examination table. She is pushing the baby with involuntary urgent force. I can see the baby's brown hair; I try to control the mother's breath to decrease the pushing power and prevent a perineumal tear; simultaneously, I put my right palm on the perineum against the bulging of the baby's head since she is unable to control the urgency of the force. The baby almost flies out through the birth canal. We lay the baby on a white cotton sheet, and I tie his umbilical cord with suture thread and cut him free.

The baby is crying hard. He is a healthy and beautiful boy, approximately 7 1/2 pounds in weight and 20 inches long. My nurse Laura takes the mother's blood pressure and pulse, which are stable. Mr. Denney wipes his wife's sweat from her brow. In several minutes, by another strong push, the afterbirth comes out in a pool of blood over the table sheet and in the basin. I examine it thoroughly, there is no defect. I massage the uterus, which contracts well and bleeding is minimal. I wrap the crying baby in a white office towel and hand him to his mother. Her face glows with happiness, already forgetting her hard labor pain, and she cries with joy. She hands the baby to her husband with mixed smiles and tears.

"You will have a little discomfort when I give you a local anesthetic for the suturing of the tear in your bottom," I warn her. After completion of the perineumal repair, Laura checks Mrs. Denney's vital signs, which are stable. I recommend that she go to the hospital, where her and her baby's condition can be observed.

"I don't have insurance to cover that. I waited to go to the hospital until the last possible minute to minimize the cost. But then it was too late to get to the hospital, so my husband brought me here. I feel good right now. The baby looks good too. If you send me home, my husband and I would greatly appreciate it," she says.

"Then I will release you to go home. I have been watching you and checking your vital signs for the last hour and a half. Probably you will be all right; but if you have any problems, let me know right away. Otherwise, you must come to the office in six weeks for a check up. This is your second baby, so you know how to take care of him. You said you were going to try breast feeding this time. You must take the baby to the pediatrician for a routine checkup with proper immunizations." I give her these instructions.

When Mr. Denney holds the baby and the mother walks out to the waiting room, the waiting people applaud with joyful smiles; some are trying to peek at the baby. Thus, the drama of our office delivery is ended. This incident is the first and the last office delivery in my practice.

Hyun A, the usual course of my day is morning surgeries followed by making hospital rounds, and office hours in the afternoon. The volume of work varies day by day, but the long hours are certain. To overcome the long hours, I contrive my own schedule for having time for myself halfway through the long day. Around lunch time, for one hour, I carry my beeper in my pocket, leaving instructions to the hospital operators as well as to the office staff not to page me unless an emergency occurs. I shall be on time at the office for my office hours; now I begin a break that restores my effectiveness and poise for the judgment and labor needed in dealing with case after case of patients.

I slip out of the noise and mass; I slide into a place where equanimity and solitude reign. All year round is pitched the lofty canopy of heaven; underneath the canopy, the universal light is ever burning; beneath the light, the cloud strata play hide-and-seek with the sun. On the earth under the canopy are the blue waters of Lake Erie; the poplar woods by the shore sing with the shore breeze all summer long, housing the thousands of birds who play a sweet concert there.

Hundreds of different flowers vaunt their beauty on the grassy bank. This is the desolate, open Sterling State Park, the place I love to go.

When I cross over the Dixie Freeway and go toward Sterling State Park, there is a winding road by the green soybean fields. Here the air is suffused with the sweet, strong scent of the wild musk rose from the thick brier thickets; pink morning glories twine and trail over the bush grove. Ancient, stately poplar trees edge the lake; a few weeping willows languidly droop at the bank, etching their green shadows on the water. Nearby, wherever the water borders on the curving pouched ground, patches of cattails and reeds flourish. Most of the time not a single boat is here; not a man walks here. But occasionally an old black couple comes in a ramshackle station wagon to sit on the picnic chairs, cast a line, and wait for the fish to bite. They look infinitely easy and happy, free of worries. Noisy flocks of seagulls are playing here, either hovering in the air or rocking on the water.

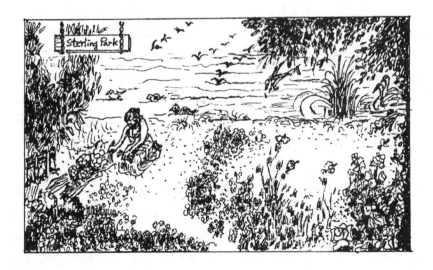

When I walk further along the bank, I see the life around me as on a stage. In the muddy water along the bank, three turtles are resting on the fallen dead trunk of a tree. The smallest one drops off into the water. The other two are basking in the hot sun, drawing out their necks fully, not stirring their heads—like mannequins in a museum display. My own neck starts to feel sore. Suddenly on the bank I see a big chestnut-shelled turtle; as soon as I see her, I halt my feet and breath and watch to see what she is doing. She plucks grasses and carries them in her mouth to hide a big hole in the center of the trail, and then she lumbers down and splashes into the water. I rush to the hole and remove the grass. I see in the recess multiple big white eggs—bigger than hen's eggs. My heart is pounding in exhilaration as though I have seized a piece of the secret of universal life. I put back a handful of the grass that the mother had used to camouflage the hole.

Sometimes my footsteps frighten the brood pheasants that nestle among the wildly grown tall grasses over the bank. They flutter away with wildly cracking cries. As I go to their nest and peek in, behind the tall grasses' wall I find they left three small eggs. Sometimes I glance at a wild duck that is brooding over her eggs behind the grassy curtain. I pretend not to notice her and stealthily pass by through the patches of blue violets. In the late spring of the mating season, the fish in the pond become frenzied, pumping up their androgens: the black backs of carps are moving and wagging and splashing and chasing along the shallow water where water weeds and cattails grow to mate and lay their eggs.

When the summer sun is too warm, the shore breeze cools me. The pale blue chicory and wild white carrots line my way on the trail. All the ponds are riotous with the reddish-purple flowers of purple loosestrife around the edges of the bank. The large, showy, pink flowers of the swamp roses invite visitors even in the distance. A bright male mallard with his green head and red neck is accompanied by his brown life mate. A flock of small black ducks, American cooters, frolic with them. A few long-legged, lonely herons or white egrets stand apart; each fixes its feet in the water and stretches its long neck like a stick.

I see the white lilies floating on the water among their spreading green leaves. The sun brightens them like unearthly flowers. At the further curve round the bank, the clearer shallow water bears the water-loving plants and turns into a partially green pond: the blue water hyacinths with curly leathery leaves, pickerel weed with white flowers, arrowhead arums with large arrowhead-shaped green leaves, water lettuces with floating leaves growing as rosettes, and sedges and rushes that seem like grasses in the water. Occasionally, black-backed carps visit there, wagging their tails. And also giant blue dragonflies and small red ones stop by for a moment and fly away repeatedly; the sunbeams glitter on their sheer wings.

In the latter part of the summer, when the pinkish-purple Canadian thistles fade into white shaggy seed balls, tiny golden finches clutch the thistles' swinging stems and peck their favorite seeds. The summer breeze puffs the seeds into the air, parachuting them like snowflakes in winter. On the grassy bank, the silverweeds' bright yellow petals are hiding and beaming in the grasses. Around another corner of the bank, yellow primroses purse their petals, unfolding only in the evening. Common milkweeds and swamp milkweeds bear their flower balls of dusky pink or bright red orange. The yellow, white or Monaco butterflies flit about, playing with the flowers rather than working. Stalks of sturdy yellow goldenrod and blue meadow asters adorn the late summer and autumnal banks. From early spring to the first frost, the banks of Lake Erie are decked continuously with a variety of wild flowers; as one flower fades away, another kind of flower comes to bloom.

When autumn comes, the green leaves on the deciduous trees to scarlet, saffron, and tawn; the tall wild grasses and green cattails stand dead in yellow brown. The red-winged blackbirds and marsh wrens wander about and claw on the cattails' lifeless stems. Their cylindrical dark-purple seed tubes burst open into the wind, sending the seeds to unknown destinations. The autumnal wind shakes the black spikes of the reeds and rustles their dry, sapless leaves. The green life of summer recedes into roots or seeds; the frosty air and bleak winds come back. Ice forms at the edge of the lake. These changes accentuate the solitude of the forlorn Sterling State Park. Knowing that next year spring shall surely come back allows birds, green plants, and men to endure the long winter.

My one-hour break at any time of year, contacting nature in solitude, refreshes me. I begin my afternoon office hours.

—16—

Case Histories

Dear Hyun A,

Gradually, year after year, more doctors come into town, and the number of patients in the hospital increases. Now anesthesiologists with anesthetists work in the Department of Anesthesia. In the OB Department, a C-section room is set up next to the labor and delivery room. Mercy and Memorial Hospitals merge and become Mercy-Memorial Hospital. The hospital care and facilities make great strides; they expand and catch up to new technology. As time and technology advance, new tools for diagnosis and treatment in my office are added and are invaluable: cryo-cautery, colposcopy, fetal monitoring, hysteroscopy, and ulrasonography.

Hyun A, no matter what tools I use or what effort and care I put into my practice, sometimes I must drink a bitter cup. Mrs. Debbie Culligan, thirty-one years old, comes to my office for secondary infertility. She has been trying to have a second baby for eight years. By laparoscopic examination, I determine that her problem is endometriosis. After over a year of hormonal therapy, which caused many side effects, finally she is pregnant. She suffers from morning sickness until the end of three months of pregnancy. Close prenatal care shows that she and her baby have grown properly up to ten days before her due day. But one morning she phones me: "Dr. Rhee, my baby is not kicking any more. I don't exactly feel sick, but sometimes I'm slightly chilly and I'm losing my appetite," she says.

"How long?"

"For the last few days."

"Why don't you come this afternoon? I'll check you," I answer. I hope she is wrong, that she may have caught cold and the baby may be quiet. However, her call gives me great uneasiness.

My nurse Laura takes her vital signs and weighs her. She has no fever, but she has lost two pounds. Her face is shaded with anxiety. I measure the fundus length with a roller ruler and listen to the fetal heart tone with an ultrasound fetoscope. I cannot find a heartbeat. My own heart throbs strongly under my rib cage. Mrs. Culligan reads my face; my face is worse than hers. Silence grows heavy in the examination room. I put transparent blue jelly on her abdomen and scan the baby with an ultrasound cable bar which shows the baby's picture on the screen by the examination table. Definitely the fetus is still, with no heart pulsation. She covers her face with her hands and sobs; I sit her up, and she leans on my shoulder, bursting out her cries. My hands are on her back, rubbing her to give her consolation. I check the cervix's pliability for the forthcoming onset of labor. I give her instructions as to what she should do and expect: "At this moment, I don't know why this has happened despite our vigilant follow up. You go home and take it easy; don't do anything strenu-

ous. I checked the mouth of your womb, which is in a favorable condition to initiate labor spontaneously. I'll give you a one-week appointment; if labor does not occur before then, you come to the
office." Mr. Culligan comes from work to pick her up.

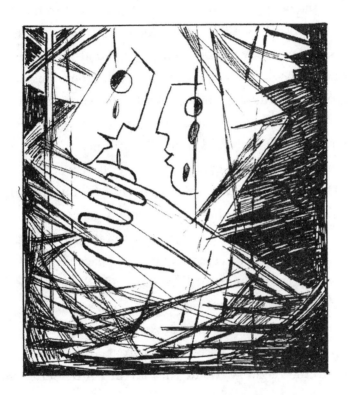

Within a week she comes to the hospital in labor and goes
through travail just as in a living baby's labor. Mr. Culligan is in the
labor room as well as the delivery room with her, which supports
her greatly. She delivers the baby in a gloomy and depressed atmosphere. No one utters a word. As soon as the baby is born, a nurse
swathes him and puts him into the bassinet. We don't know if we
should show the baby—he is terribly disfigured, with the collapsed
skull of the dead fetus, peeling skin, and discoloration of the entire

skin. How would Mr. and Mrs. Culligan react to that sight? She is calmly sniffling and wiping her eyes and nose; he holds the sides of her head with his hands, occasionally giving his kisses on her brow. They say they don't want to see their baby, but they would like to know the baby's gender.

After the delivery is over, Mrs. Culligan is sent to the recovery room on the postpartum floor. I check the baby with the OB nurses. The baby is male and weights about seven pounds; he is well developed with no obvious abnormalities or cord around his neck. The baby is baptized with water on his brow in the name of Jesus Christ. His parents do not want to consent to an autopsy. Even though the parents refused to see him, I think of this: once the baby is taken away from here, they can never see him. They have worked so hard to have this baby for so long and have carried him for nine months; they may not be able to forget him, and he might haunt them for a lifetime. But if they see and touch the baby, even though his appearance is grotesque, they may be able to let him go peacefully. I discuss this with the OB nurses who helped with Mrs. Culligan's labor and delivery. I believe that older nurses have more experience in life's tragedies and have better solutions. They weigh my suggestion, saying, "There is nothing to lose in asking the parents once more."

I go to the recovery room. They are in a little better mood. I talk about the baby's weight and the result of my examination. They are pleased to hear that there was nothing abnormal. I offer them the chance to see the baby, with my reasons for it. After several minutes of decision making, summoning their courage, they say, "Yes, Dr. Rhee, we would like to see him."

Soon they are brought to the delivery area where the baby is placed, and the nurses show them the baby. They bravely face the baby lying still in the white swath, and they touch him; eventually they let him go, giving him their blessings.

The father takes his son to bury him by his grandfather. The mother is dismissed from the hospital in three days.

Before she leaves she says, "Dr. Rhee, thank you for all your help in conception, during pregnancy, and in delivery, and for helping us go through our ordeals."

One year later, they try to have another baby, and they bring forth a healthy, crying son who brings them great joy.

Hyun A, as medical technology advances, more and more things become possible as though men walked on the moon: the doctors transplant one man's heart or liver to another man; a man's sperm or a woman's ova can be frozen and still be alive; the doctors can grow a fetus in an incubation tube. By virtue of such scientific progress, Mr. and Mrs. Goldon have their babies. If they had lived before this century, they could never have seen their children or even dreamed of having them.

Scott and Betty Goldon come to my office for primary infertility. They have been married for ten years and have been trying to have a baby all that time. Following an extensive infertility workup for both husband and wife, I find that it is necessary for her to have auxiliary hormonal therapy to aid ovulation. For that purpose, clomid is used; she conceives a baby. Before she takes the medicine, I warn the couple of the possibility of multiple pregnancies. At the end of the third month, the ultrasound screen at the office shows that she is going to have twin babies. The couple do not want to know the babies' gender. However, after seeing the two babies moving and seeing their little hearts thumping, their excitement is doubled.

"Oh my gosh! It is incredible!" "It's a miracle! Unbelievable" both Mr. and Mrs. Goldon exclaim, holding each other.

I give them instructions and warnings about the problems prone to occur during a multiple pregnancy. Premature labor is far more prevalent in a twin than in a single pregnancy.

Therefore, the further the pregnancy advances, the more bed rest is needed. With a blush of excitement, they withdraw from the examination room, carrying their twins' pictures.

Mrs. Goldon carries her babies well throughout her pregnancy except for her saying, "Dr. Rhee, I can put my meal tray upon my stomach!" She comes to the hospital at thirty-eight weeks in labor. Again she and her husband are aware of possible complications. Initially her labor progresses normally and the first baby's position and the mother's condition are all right, but if the second baby will not turn, I will have to deliver by a C-section. Therefore, Mrs. Goldon can take nothing by mouth, and a technician draws blood to prepare for the cross-matching of blood.

After eight hours of labor, Mrs. Goldon delivers the first baby, a healthy girl who weights 5 lbs. 4 oz. About seven minutes later, as the white, glistening, bulging bag shows up, I break it with an amniotic hook and am splattered by gushing fluid. The second baby slides out through the birth canal; the baby boy is crying hard. He weights 4 lbs. 3 oz. The OB nurses put white cotton caps on the babies' heads to preserve their body heat and wrap them with baby blankets. They hand the babies to their parents: one to the mother, the other to the father. The delivery room is filled with joyous clamor mingling the two babies' crying, laughter, and exclamations: "Look at his long black hair! A big mouth! A big nose just like his father!"

Mr. Goldon has been with his wife throughout the entire course of her labor, and also he has attended her in the delivery room. He has supported her morale and has shared in the joy of holding the newborn babies. In general, a father in the labor and delivery room not only benefits the couple, but it greatly decreases the doctors' and nurses' work loads physically and emotionally. Indeed, a father has a right to share the joy of the babies' birth because he and his wife have created their babies together.

As life has both sweet and bitter edges, the medical practice has both such edges.

One moment in my medical practice has both the bitter and the sweet. It is the height of spring. On the bare magnolia trees and on the forsythia bushes, the brilliant blossoms are yellow and pink everywhere. Near my office on North Macomb Street, the maple trees bearred buds on the black branches. The warmer air after the cold winter spawns all life on the earth. In this season, during the middle of my afternoon office hours, I see a patient who most likely has ovarian cancer.

The patient comes to see me because she has recently noticed abdominal discomfort, lower back pain associated with indigestion, and a sense of bloating—the actual feeling of her stomach swelling. She is a white female, divorced, fifty-four years old. She has had one pregnancy and one child, who was born thirty-two years ago. Fifteen years ago she had an abdominal hysterectomy owing to irregular vaginal bleeding and a benign fibroid uterine tumor. At that time she was thirty-nine years old, so her gynecologist left her one ovary to provide proper female hormones. Until five years ago, she visited her gynecologist regularly for her routine check up without any problems. But her doctor died, and for the last five years she has not visited a gynecologist.

I examine her. She appears distressed and slightly pale. Her vital signs and breast examination are within normal range. Her lungs sound clear, her liver is enlarged, and by percussion on her abdomen, I definitely feel the fluid waves. The pelvic examination shows no abnormal lesions in the vagina or vulva. During the vaginal examination I feel an undefinable hard mass, and also there is a tender, larger, vaguely palpable mass in the left pelvic cavity.

The next day she is admitted to the hospital and is tested with a variety of blood work, x-ray, and sonogram studies. After collecting all the results, under the tentative diagnosis of an advanced ovarian cancer, I do an exploratory laparatomy on her. She obviously has a left ovarian cancer which has spread to all the adjacent organs—rectum, liver, omentum, and diaphragm. During surgery, I order a frozen biopsy—which proves the malignant adenocarcinoma of the ovary—and I remove the ovarian cancer mass as completely as I can. She tolerates the surgery well. After the surgery is finished, I discuss Mrs. Cooper's present condition and further treatment with her daughter and son-in-law. I ask her daughter whether I should tell her mother the bad news now or wait and let the daughter tell her mother herself. The daughter, Debbie Hoffman, says her mother is very intelligent and already realizes she may have some sort of fatal disease. "I think it is better to tell my mother the truth; then she can prepare properly for the rest of her short life and face her final days. I think, Dr. Rhee, that you must tell her all about her situation and further treatment plan because she trusts you more than anyone else."

And so on the third day after surgery, after I check the wound and change the dressing, I explain her condition to Mrs. Cooper. "The pathological study proves that you have definite ovarian cancer which has already spread to other organs. You need further treatment. For that purpose, I will refer you to a gynecological oncologist in the University of Michigan Hospital."

She at first bursts into sobs and then tries to restrain her emotion. Her recovery from the surgery is smooth, but her morale is dejected. Then much to my surprise, on the sixth day after surgery when I enter her room making rounds, I find her putting makeup on her thin face. Her hair is nicely combed and pinned on the back of her head with a black bow; she wears a long, light pink nightgown and fancy pink slippers. Above all, her despondent expression is transformed into a glow of bloom, as if she is a different person. Her morning greeting is cheery, and vigorous. "Wow! What's going on today, Mrs. Cooper?" I ask. She does not stumble over her words.

"Dr. Rhee, this morning my ex-husband will come to see me! Yesterday he called me and said he would like to see me if I would allow him to do so. So I said all right," she says, smiling brightly. "He and I divorced after five years of marriage when our daughter was three years old—I never heard a single word of hers condemning him. After I divorced, I went to Michigan State University to major in English Literature; I obtained a bachelor's and a master's degree in English from the same university; I became an English teacher at the high school in my home town. I never married again, but he married another woman and had two sons. I saw him last on my daughter's wedding day."

From that day on, her animated spirit and positive attitude are unimaginable in a patient who knows she is in the terminal stage of a fatal disease. Following discharge from the hospital, she goes to the University of Michigan Hospital. When I see her at the four weeks' follow-up at my office, her wound is healed well and her swollen abdomen and general condition are not getting drastically worse, even though she looks anemic. She still has her good cheer and happy glow.

"Dr. Rhee, can I show you my wedding ring?" she asks. For a moment her words puzzle me. I am unable to respond to her. She proudly and happily puts out her left hand and shows me a large, glittering diamond on her ring finger. "I have to believe that ring," I say to myself.

"Scott, my husband, told me he truly loves me. Since four years ago, after his second wife died in a car accident, he has been living alone because his two sons are married. When he heard about my illness through Debbie, he had to come to see me. He asked if he could take care of me.

He said that if I allow him to marry me, he would like to marry at once and live with me. But to avoid any misconceptions concerning his love for me, he wanted to legally confirm that all my property will go to Debbie after I die. And he showed me his sincerity and deep love even though I am in difficulty. So I married him. Now Scott and I live in a true second revitalized honeymoon."

She says that he is here in the waiting room. And she assures me that she is following up the radiation therapy schedule at the University of Michigan.

One year later I learn that she died happily and peacefully in her husband's arms at the University of Michigan Hospital. Her husband took care of the funeral, and he moved out of the house, bequeathing it to their daughter.

The terminal stage of ovarian cancer brought back their love to Mr. and Mrs. Cooper. Whatever disrupted their love and family for so many long years, they forgave each other and started a new life filled with unconditional love, and then they fulfilled their true purpose of life. There is no more beautiful and powerful thing in the world than *Love*.

Hyun A, in the middle of the night, from the depth of sleep, often I have to get up and go to the hospital to deliver a baby. This is not an easy or pleasant thing to do. That's why most interns do not choose to be obstetricians. They know that babies often come at night. No one knows exactly why, yet people theorize comically or logically. They say babies are made at night, so they must come at night; or they say that the full moon influences the onset of labor, owing to the moon's gravity that initiates labor as the moon controls the river's tide, waxing and waning. Night-delivered babies bring me sometimes hard life, but special benefits, too. If the babies had not called for my help at night, my senses would have been dulled or would have rusted away in bed while sleeping.

The features of night are not as scary as they appear. You might think that night is pitch dark; everything lies cowering under that dark, monstrous mask. My babies show me the different aspects of night. They are the night's beauty and wonder. In the dead of one bitter night, after delivering a baby, I head for home. The road is cleared of snow, but it's piled and frozen on the sidewalks and ground. The air is cutting and crisp; tiny flickering stars are on its farthest dome, and the white Milky Way sweeps as a long white trail. The white fluorescent full moon seems like a single giant universal street-light lighting up the sleeping earth. Her perfect beauty glows through the dark bare branches of ancient oaks around our house on Riverview Road.

I get out of the car, crunching the frozen snow, and reach the porch door. However, something behind is pulling me; I turn around and walk back to the driveway, crunching on over the snow, gazing up at the high stars and the moon. Strangely, this noise does not shatter the silence. The stars are calling me to stay with them and to communicate with them for a little while. How can we do so? We are millions, billions, or trillions of miles away from each other; reaching them even with the speed of light would take years. But I am experiencing the fact that through our imagination, there are no obstacles of distance. Our imagination is faster than the speed of light. The more I gaze up at the night sky, the more its beauty is revealed: it is reserved, calm, lofty, majestic, grand, and mystical.

The night sky shows me that I am tiny, like a particle of dust in this universe. It reminds me that beyond my world there are measureless worlds and suns and planets. The night sky expands my mind from a particle of dust to the infinity of universal space. When I get into the bedroom, the round moon behind the black oak's branches shines on my bed through the veil of shades.

Thus, babies reward me by somehow awakening my buried sensibilities in return for my helping them come into this world.

Hyun A, one later evening in mid January, I am called by a labor and delivery room nurse and told that a baby will soon be ready to deliver. This is a baby that the mother and father have wanted for a long time. They had an infertility problem and have gone through many surgical and endocrinological procedures to conceive this child. It is a cold night; the presence of wind is hardly noticeable. Thick snow-holding clouds obscure the entire dark sky.

At the hospital, I check the patient; the baby is not yet ready. I stay at the doctor's oncall room on the third floor of the west wing and look out through the window. Small fleecy snowflakes begin to fill the vast, vacant space above the ground, dancing in the window light; these flakes look like moving particles in the wintry air. They are not plummeting down or speeding up, but gracefully, with rhythm, they are whirling, spinning, and flying as if with acrobatic wings. I wonder, why do they fly in the air rather than fall when there is no wind to whirl and spin them? The flakes answer, "We are extremely thin and light, all but weightless. Therefore we are soundless and flying and dancing." Some touch the towering evergreen spruces and firs and pines on the lighted hospital parking grounds. Some come to the window, knocking mutely. Like angels, they seem to try to whisper to me their heavenly secret of the place from which they come. Then they bounce back from the window and fly away to an unknown destination. Be it ever so fleeting a moment, the heavenly angels have left me bliss and have awakened my dormant spirit to write.

If I let this overwhelming moment pass without recording it in any form—a poem, an essay, a diary, a song—what good would it be except to myself? When I die, nothing would be left to our children and their children as a legacy. On the other hand, if I do try, my overpowering moment of thought and emotion will last as my very spirit. I may be able to touch other souls as these snow angels have touched mine. From that day on, I have kept writing, whether it be of great significance or of little significance. I feel that every man has his own position and his own talent in this universe. A little man may be as important and authoritative as a great man. Meager or imperfect as his work may be, if he did his best and nothing more can be done than what he accomplished, it would be sufficient to say, "His work is significant." He has created, with his soul, a form of creative work that represents himself. In this way, I rationalize my need to write in my poor, stumbling English as well as in my own Korean tongue.

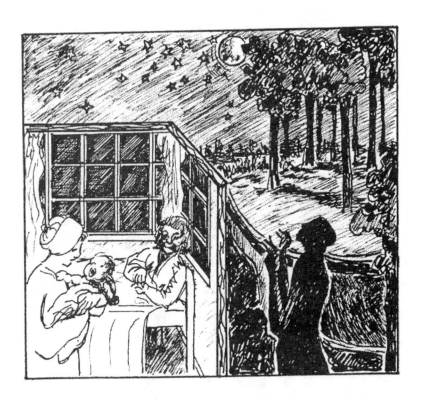

Shortly after, the snow clears. I deliver a healthy baby girl who weighs eight pounds, without complications. Hyun A, you wouldn't believe what the mother tells me when I lift up the naked baby and show it to her who is still lying in pain on the delivery table.

"Dr. Rhee, we are naming her after you: Sunny Laura Ginsburg!"

Hyun A, don't we have the best profession? I will remember this moment always as one touched by a shaft of sacred light. All the labor, all the sacrifice, all the years of study seem to culminate in this one transcendent moment. For I am a doctor. I am here to help to bring life into the world. And I will write about how this came to be.

—17—

My Creed

Dear Hyun A,

You and I have the same profession, and so I am comfortable—actually glad—to say what I think about my role as a doctor because you can understand my meaning. I am sure you have your own physician's creed. Mine is this:

Hyun A, I believe that medicine is a vocation of healing art. The vocation requires physicians to be men of integrity. Regardless of whether the patients be old or young, rich or poor, physicians are here to help all the sick and to help men from getting sick. The vocation requires that physicians not only be helpers but at the same time be humanists to share and to feel their patients' pain and misery. For physicians are directly linked to a patient's life and death. Therefore, a physician must have the qualities of compassion, kindness, and sincerity.

189

I think physicians are privileged because they have the special knowledge and skill that allows them to help and to heal. Every physician goes through many years of painstaking study and training—the longest period of any field—to become a physician. At the end of his struggle is the power to change a patient's life.

I think physicians must be competent in knowledge, skill, and ethics in their work. In addition, they must constantly keep up with new knowledge and techniques to give their patients the best possible care.

Often I am confronted with hard times; for example, in the middle of the night I have to wake up and go to the hospital to deliver babies or to perform emergency surgeries. After my long hours of daytime work without much rest, it is not an easy thing to do. Sometimes I must make a difficult decision. I must try to be right. At such times I simply question myself:

> What if I or one of my family were that patient? What would I desire my doctor to do for me?

> Definitely, I would want him to be competent, skillful, and knowledgeable so that I can trust him and rely on him for the treatment of my illness. I would want him to show me kindness, sincerity, and compassion for my pain. Let him not harm me, exploit me, or mislead me.

This creed clears away most of my obstacles and sheds the light of conscience on my duty as a physician. When I follow this creed, I rarely see an alternative road to derail me from my vocation or from the Hippocratic oath.

I know you understand this, my beloved Hyun A. And I am so proud of you. For you, too, are a doctor.

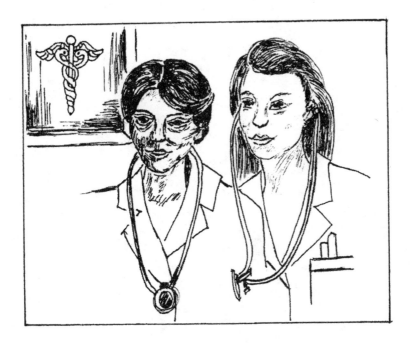

Passing the Torch

The flame
of my torch that I now
pass to you is the crystallization
of all my body, mind, and soul as love,
strength, goodness, and an unending quest
for knowledge. It will abide in you, giving you a shaft of
light when you grope in the dark, offering calm comfort while
you are in despair, and stirring your inner strength when you
think that you have failed. Hyun A, I have an unwavering
faith that in your lifetime you will create your own torch
to add to mine—brighter and mightier than your
mom's—to hand on your own children.
And your children will then hand
theirs to their children.
Just as the Olympic
fire of ancient
Greece is still
burning in the
hearts of
mankind, my
spirit in flame
abides in your
blood, and yours
in your children.
Like the
unending
chapters of
generations,
they burn
on
forever!
Your mom